Handbook for EMS Medical Directors

March 2012

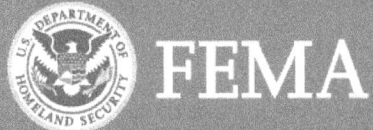 FEMA

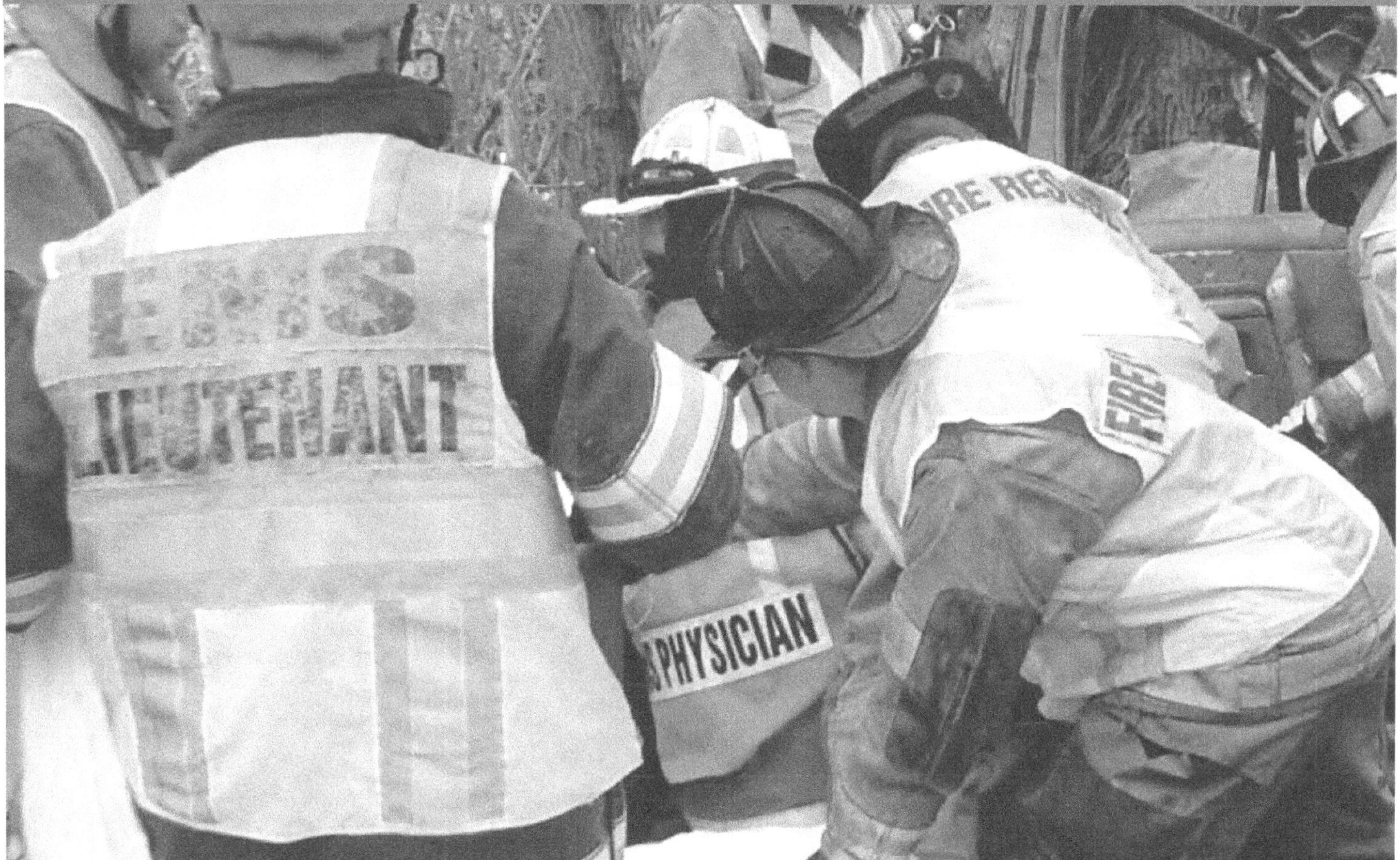

U.S. Fire Administration

Mission Statement

We provide National leadership to foster a solid foundation for our fire and emergency services stakeholders in prevention, preparedness, and response.

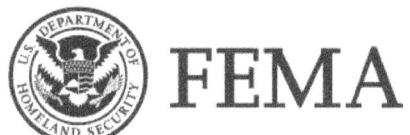 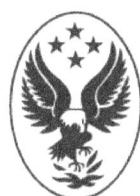

Preface

Colleagues:

The Department of Homeland Security (DHS) Office of Health Affairs (OHA) and the U.S. Fire Administration (USFA) are pleased to deliver this *Handbook for EMS Medical Directors* of local departments and agencies involved in emergency medical services (EMS) response.

Medical directors provide critical oversight and medical direction to ensure that effective emergency medical care is provided to millions of patients throughout the United States. In addition to providing medical oversight and direction, EMS medical directors support EMS personnel and first responders through training, protocol development, and resource deployment advice. This handbook provides a baseline overview of key roles and responsibilities to assist current and prospective medical directors in performing their important missions.

On behalf of the U.S. DHS, we thank you for your service to the Nation's EMS.

Sincerely yours,

Alexander G. Garza, M.D., M.P.H.
Assistant Secretary for Health Affairs and
Chief Medical Officer

Ernest Mitchell, Jr.
U.S. Fire Administrator

Table of Contents

Acknowledgements

The *Handbook for EMS Medical Directors* was developed by the International Association of Fire Chiefs (IAFC) as part of a Cooperative Agreement with the Department of Homeland Security (DHS), Federal Emergency Management Agency (FEMA), U.S. Fire Administration (USFA), and was supported by DHS, Office of Health Affairs (OHA). The IAFC Emergency Medical Services (EMS) Section provided oversight in the development of the handbook.

A project team representing EMS stakeholder groups worked together to develop, contribute, and author the handbook. The following individuals are extended the greatest amount of appreciation for their expertise, effort, and dedication throughout the handbook development process:

Edward Dickinson, MD, NREMT-P, FACEP
National Association of EMS Physicians (NAEMSP)

George Lindbeck, MD
National Association of State EMS Officials
(NASEMSO)

Chief Gary Ludwig, MS, EMT-P
International Association of Fire Chiefs (IAFC)

Lori Moore-Merrell, DrPH
International Association of Fire Fighters (IAFF)

Chief Mary Beth Michos (ret.), MS
Chief Administrative and Operations Officer
International Association of Fire Chiefs (IAFC)

Victoria Lee, MPA
Program Manager
International Association of Fire Chiefs (IAFC)

Battalion Chief Jennie L. Collins, NREMT-P
Lead Technical Writer

Lieutenant James H. Logan, BS, EMT-P
Technical Writer

Richard W. Patrick, MS, CFO, EMT-P
U.S. Department of Homeland Security (DHS),
Office of Health Affairs (OHA)

Bill Troup, MBA
Fire Program Specialist
U.S. Fire Administration (USFA)
National Fire Data Center (NFDC)

Chief Ed Plaugher (ret.), BS, EFO
Assistant Executive Director
International Association of Fire Chiefs (IAFC)

Melissa Milan, MD
Technical Writer

In addition to the project team, many industry professionals contributed time, information, and efforts to aid in the production of this handbook. Industry stakeholder groups reviewed and provided feedback during the handbook's production and their efforts are greatly appreciated. Listed below are the stakeholder groups and their representatives who reviewed the handbook.

American Ambulance Association (AAA)
Jeffrey M. Goodloe, MD, NREMT-P, FACEP

American College of Emergency Physicians (ACEP)
David J. Schoenwetter, DO, FACEP

International Association of EMS Chiefs (IAEMSC)
John Peruggia, BSHS, EFO, EMT-P

International Association of Fire Chiefs (IAFC)
Gary Ludwig, MS, EMT-P

IAFC's Safety, Health and Survival Section
Ed Nied, MST, NREMT-P

International Association of Fire Fighters (IAFF)
Lori Moore-Merrell, DrPH

National Association of Emergency
Medical Technicians (NAEMT)
Jason Kodat, MD, EMT-P

National Association of EMS Educators (NAEMSE)
Angel Clark Burba, MS, NREMT-P, NCEE

National Association of EMS Physicians (NAEMSP)
Edward Dickinson, MD, NREMT-P, FACEP

National Association of State EMS Officials
(NASEMSO)
George Lindbeck, MD

National EMS Management Association (NEMSMA)
Jerry Allison, MD, MS

National Fire Protection Association (NFPA)
Ken Holland, FF/EMT-P, BA, MBA/PA

National Volunteer Fire Council (NVFC)
Ken Knipper

U.S. Department of Homeland Security (DHS),
Office of Health Affairs (OHA)
Sandy Bogucki, MD, Ph.D., FACEP

U.S. Department of Homeland Security (DHS),
Office of Health Affairs (OHA)
Michael Zanker, MD
Senior Medical Associate

U.S. Department of Homeland Security (DHS),
Office of Health Affairs (OHA)
Michael Zanker, MD, FACEP,
Senior Medical Officer

U.S. Department of Transportation
National Highway Traffic Safety Administration
(NHTSA) Office of EMS
Drew Dawson

Other technical input was received from:

Franklin D. Pratt, M.D., MPHTM, FACEP
Medical Director, Los Angeles County (CA)
Fire Department

Doug Wolfberg of Page, Wolfberg, and Wirth, LLC

The project team and sponsoring agencies extend their appreciation for the professional support and cooperation provided during the review process. The efforts of the project team, contributors, and authors will aid in the education of those who read the handbook and will result in improved understanding of the multifaceted role of an EMS agency medical director.

Introduction

The position of an emergency medical services (EMS) agency medical director allows the opportunity for a physician to become engaged in the unique and ever-evolving realm of out-of-hospital care, a clinical practice offering a distinct set of challenges, and rewarding impacts in improving a community's emergency medical care abilities. For most, the driving force behind the desire to become an EMS agency medical director stems from a deep passion for helping patients in times of marked acute medical need whenever and wherever the need appears. Yet, understanding the nuances involved in the oversight and direction of an EMS agency requires specialized knowledge, skills, and abilities beyond the typical curriculum of emergency medicine or alternative acute care medical practices. It is for this precise reason that EMS has been recently recognized by the American Board of Medical Specialties as a formal physician subspecialty.

The purpose of this handbook is to provide assistance to both new and experienced medical directors as they strive to provide the highest quality of out-of-hospital emergency medical care to their communities and foster excellence within their agencies. The handbook will provide the new medical director with a fundamental orientation to the roles that define the position of the medical director while providing the experienced medical director with a useful reference tool. The handbook will explore the nuances found in the EMS industry—a challenge to describe in generalities due to the tremendous amount of diversity among EMS agencies and systems across the Nation. The handbook does not intend to serve as an operational medical practice document, but seeks to identify and describe the critical elements associated with the position.

EMS medical direction is a multidimensional activity that includes the direction and oversight of administrative, operational, educational, and clinical actions related to patient care activities. The medical director is an integral leader in an EMS agency and will serve as the interface between the agency and the medical community. The medical director must have a collaborative and cooperative approach to working with the EMS agency, as there are many who will work in concert to ensure the agency is functioning optimally.

The EMS workforce is a diverse, creative, committed, and often very street-savvy group of providers. The medical director can be most effective by meshing the physician passions for patient beneficence, scientific discovery, ethical practices, and professional development to the enthusiasm and dedication within the EMS culture. Achieving success as a medical director depends on many things. Inherent among them is a tremendous amount of motivation, willingness to learn while simultaneously teaching, and enacting solid leadership skills, all while reinforcing the roles of patient advocate, mentor, and coach. The successful medical director is equally analytical and resourceful. The medical director must focus on how to improve their agency and the service that it delivers on a continual basis. Involvement with this aspect of emergency care can be extremely rewarding, challenging, as well as personally and professional fulfilling. Physicians electing to pursue the role of a medical director are to be commended for their dedication and critical position they will hold in the public safety and health care arenas.

The handbook's chapters identify and discuss the components of an EMS agency and its agency stakeholders, the position of a medical director, and the medical director's role in agency oversight. The handbook contains appendices that include

- medical director's checklist;

- glossary;

- acronym guide;

- sample agreement of service documents;

- sample liability insurance documents;

- industry regulations and standards; and

- sample performance measures.

These reference items will aid in a physician's understanding of the general role, needs, and requirements for the medical director position.

The EMS Agency and Its Stakeholders

Overview

The emergency medical services (EMS) system describes a continuum of care beginning with initial contact and response through patient care and transport to an appropriate receiving facility. EMS also has grown in its involvement in other areas of out-of-hospital care including disaster and mass casualty planning and injury prevention. The "EMS Agenda for the Future" describes prehospital medicine as the practice of providing emergency care that is remote from a health-care facility, in all of its complexities.[1]

An EMS agency is a coordinated arrangement of personnel, equipment, and facilities organized to respond to medical emergencies regardless of cause. Since the care of patients in the EMS arena also includes those patients needing movement between health-care facilities (e.g., hospital to nursing or rehabilitation facility) and not just their entry into the health-care system due to an emergency, the term out-of-hospital care is also used to describe the EMS environment.

EMS History

EMS can trace its roots to humble beginnings and unlikely sponsors. During the early to mid-20th century, funeral homes operated the majority of vehicles used for "EMS." The funeral homes' hearses could accommodate the need to transport a body on a stretcher and served a dual purpose by either taking the dead to the funeral home or the living to the hospital. For the most part, funeral home personnel were not trained in patient care and could do little more than rapidly drive the living to the hospital and hope their condition would not deteriorate during the trip.

Early EMS agencies, commonly called rescue squads, developed in an inconsistent manner and widely varied across America's communities, especially following the end of World War II. Military campaigns have been a considerable source for many of the advancements in the civilian out-of-hospital environment. On the battleground, there was an emphasis to rapidly treat and move the wounded soldier to a treatment area. Equipment designed for the battleground quickly became adapted into the out-of-hospital environment. World War II saw the birth of the combat medic who could administer medications such as morphine and plasma in the field, serving as the original model for advanced life support (ALS) in the civilian world. The rapid movement of wounded through the use of helicopters during the Korean and Vietnam Wars was also replicated in the civilian environment.

However, there was a dearth of any standards, a void of training programs, and sporadic availability of equipment. This all began to change when the National Academy of Sciences produced a report titled "Accidental Death and Disability: The Neglected Disease of Modern Society" in 1966. This publication called attention to the poor condition of emergency medical care in America by focusing on roadway trauma and deaths. Reacting to the initial link between vehicular-related trauma and inadequate EMS care, President Johnson signed the National Traffic and Motor Vehicle Safety Act of 1966. This law focused on the development of standards for highway accident victims and served as the foundation to address the fundamental deficiencies in EMS agencies. When President Johnson signed the National Traffic and Motor Vehicle Safety Act of 1966 and Federal funding became available, EMS systems quickly developed across the United States.

The Highway Safety Act of 1966 created a new Federal agency within the National Highway Safety Bureau, the predecessor of the National Highway Traffic Safety Administration (NHTSA). NHTSA was responsible for the development and implementation of EMS legislation, training standards, and agency funding that was allocated to States, regions, and locales to support EMS agencies.[2] Parallel to NHTSA's work, pioneering EMS physicians in geographically diverse areas such as Seattle (Dr. Leonard Cobb and Dr. Michael Copass),

Los Angeles (Dr. Michael Criley), New York City (Dr. Sheldon Jacobson), Columbus (Dr. James Warren), and Miami (Dr. Eugene Nagel) mentored and created a new level of sophisticated professional for out-of-hospital emergency medical care, what we now commonly refer to as the "paramedic." In the next few years, textbooks were created to support these new training curricula, reflecting an expanded scope of services to address acute medical illness as well as trauma.

In pursuit of establishing uniform training and examination standards, the National Registry of Emergency Medical Technicians (NREMT) was founded in 1970. The NREMT created a national certification agency for those individuals involved in the delivery of EMS. Mainstream media attention for EMS was gained in the early 1970s when Hollywood brought the television show "Emergency!" into American homes. The television show experienced widespread popularity and greatly contributed to improving the public's knowledge and attitude toward the value and importance of EMS, not to mention recruiting a generation of EMS providers who continue to be active in field practice, education, and administration.

It was in 1971 that an individual by the name of James O. Page, working for the Los Angeles County Fire Department, was assigned to coordinate the countywide implementation of one of the Nation's first paramedic rescue services. Jim Page served as technical consultant and writer for "Emergency!" and later founded the "Journal of Emergency Medical Services" (JEMS) publication. At the time of his untimely death, he was a retired fire chief and was serving as publisher emeritus of JEMS and "FireRescue Magazine," while also a partner in the national EMS law firm of Page, Wolfberg, and Wirth. Jim Page is easily recognized as one of the most influential individuals in the development of EMS.

The EMS System Act of 1973 (Public Law 93-154) was passed by Congress and provided funding for several hundred EMS systems across the Nation. The EMS System Act defined an EMS system and its essential components:

> "[An EMS system] provides for the arrangement of personnel, facilities, and equipment for the effective and coordinated delivery of health care services in an appropriate geographical area under emergency conditions (occurring either as a result of the patient's condition or of natural disasters or similar situations) and which is administered by a public or nonprofit private entity which has the authority and the resources to provide effective administration of the system."[3]

The EMS System Act identified 14 critical components of an EMS system:

1. Integration into the health-care system.

2. EMS research.

3. Legislation and regulation.

4. System finances.

5. Human resources.

6. Medical direction.

7. Education systems.

8. Public education.

9. Prevention.

10. Public access.

11.   Communication systems.

12.   Clinical care.

13.   Information systems.

14.   Evaluation.[4]

In 1979, emergency medicine became recognized as a specialty by the American Medical Association (AMA) and the American Board of Medical Specialties (ABMS). The AMA also recognized the emergency medical technician (EMT)/Paramedic as an allied health occupation. During the same time period, the first national standard for paramedic training was developed and professional associations for EMTs were formed.[5] One of these professional associations was the National Association of Emergency Medical Technicians (NAEMT) which is the largest professional association for EMS practitioners today.

The early 1980s brought continued efforts to standardized testing for EMS providers. The American fire service had recognized the value of EMS delivery and a preponderance of fire departments had integrated some level of EMS care in their delivery model. In 1981, direct Federal funding established by the Highway Safety Act of 1966 was switched to State block grants. The block grants were not strictly tied to EMS system development which resulted in some States electing to divert the funding to other public health initiatives judged to be more pressing. EMS systems across the Nation continued to develop inconsistently due to the wide variability among the State EMS offices and funding availability.[6] In 1985, the National Association of EMS Physicians (NAEMSP) was formed, recognizing the importance of physician involvement in EMS systems.

In the early 1990s, attention turned to improving several initiatives that were introduced in the previous decades. One example involved the three-digit emergency number, 9-1-1. While 9-1-1 was created in the 1960s, its widespread adoption and appropriate use became a focus of public education campaigns in the early 1990s. Trauma system development began in the 1960s and experienced further growth during the 1990s with emphasis on the development of comprehensive trauma systems that matched patient needs with specialized, regionalized resources. EMS managers also recognized the need to perform EMS system strategic planning to further integrate EMS into the health-care system. EMS became increasingly recognized as an important component in the continuum of health care, rather than an external system that merely delivered patients to the doorstep of the traditional health-care system. Forward thinkers began to realize that patient care could be optimized if systems were designed to include strategies for patient care beginning with their first contact with the EMS system.

Another landmark EMS-related publication was produced in 1996. NHTSA and the Department of Health and Human Services' (HHS's) Health Resources and Services Administration published a Federally funded consensus paper titled "EMS Agenda for the Future." This publication strived to establish a common vision and roadmap for the continued development of EMS systems. This roadmap was applicable to all levels of EMS agencies at the national, State, and local levels. The paper stated an overall vision for future EMS systems:

> "Emergency Medical Services (EMS) of the future will be community-based health management that is fully integrated with the overall health care system. It will have the ability to identify and modify illness and injury risks, provide acute illness and injury care and follow-up, and contribute to treatment of chronic conditions and community health monitoring. This new entity will be developed from redistribution of existing health care resources and will be integrated with other health care providers and public health and public safety agencies. It will improve community health and result in a more appropriate use of acute health care resources. EMS will remain the public's emergency medical safety net."[7]

In 2000, NHTSA released a followup report to "EMS Agenda for the Future." The new report was titled "The EMS Education Agenda for the Future: A Systems Approach." This report identified the need to develop an educational certification and licensure system that would achieve national consistency for entry-level EMS personnel.

"The EMS Education Agenda for the Future" identified the need to have an EMS education system which integrated five major components:

1.   National EMS Core Content.

2.   National EMS Scope of Practice Model.

3.   National EMS Education Standards.

4.   National EMS Certification.

5.   National EMS Education Program Accreditation.[8]

While EMS can celebrate numerous and extensive successes, EMS systems remain fragmented, overburdened, and underfunded as identified in the 2006 Institute of Medicine's (IOM's) report titled "Emergency Medical Services at the Crossroads."[9] The IOM report examined a variety of issues affecting the delivery of EMS and recognized the extent of fragmentation in the Nation's EMS systems that add complexity and variability in how EMS is delivered. The key areas impacting EMS systems were identified as:

•   insufficient coordination;

•   disparities in response times;

•   uncertain quality of care;

•   lack of readiness for disasters;

•   divided professional identity; and

•   limited evidence base that support current EMS practices.[10]

The IOM report called for improvements through a series of recommendations so that EMS systems could evolve into highly coordinated and accountable systems that functioned on a shared regional basis versus operating independently or in a vacuum. The committee's findings and recommendations have broad categories of:

•   Federal lead agency;

•   system finance;

•   regionalization;

•   national standards for training and credentialing;

•   medical direction and EMS physician subspecialization;

•   coordination;

•   communications and data systems;

•   air medical services;

- accountability;

- disaster preparedness;

- research; and

- achieving the vision.

For more information on any of the mentioned publications, the following website provides information and links to the documents: www.ems.gov/

The Modern EMS System

The modern EMS system consists of those organizations, individuals, facilities, and equipment that are required to ensure timely and medically-appropriate responses to each request for prehospital care and medical transportation. Each State, community, and agency has a distinct history and culture with respect to the EMS system. The medical director needs to understand the various requirements, culture, and the unique relationship between each agency and local and State government, as well as the relationships between providers and leadership within the agency.

Within the United States, EMS personnel treat nearly 20 million patients a year with many of these patients experiencing complicated medical or traumatic events.[11] The response, care, and transport of these patients require considerable knowledge, skills, and abilities (KSAs) on the part of the provider. The out-of-hospital environment presents numerous challenges to these skilled providers and to the agencies that support their operations.

The National EMS Scope of Practice Model identifies what procedures an EMS provider is authorized to perform by the level of provider certification or licensure. However, the National EMS Scope of Practice Model is not accepted by all States. In States where the National EMS Scope of Practice Model is not accepted, there may be other governmental authorities (State, regional, or local) who establish and define the scope of practice (specific medical procedures and interventions which may be performed) for EMS providers.

While the scope of practice defines the medical procedures and interventions that a provider is legally authorized to perform, it does not identify the standard of care. The standard of care within the EMS industry is established by identifying the level of care provided by equally trained personnel given the same situation. At the provider's agency level, the medical director needs to work cooperatively as part of the agency's leadership to establish the patient care culture through the implementation of policies, procedures and protocols, training, continuing education, and continuous quality improvement programs.

EMS personnel are unique health-care professionals in that they typically provide medical care in the out-of-hospital setting following their EMS agency's protocols and procedures, as approved by their medical director. Medical direction is a critical component in all aspects of an EMS agency's operations. A medical director may establish local protocols or assimilate regional or State structured protocols for use in their agency. Protocols are written medical standards for EMS practice, as well as the expected patient care procedures to be performed in a variety of situations. The latitude that a medical director may have in writing and establishing their own patient care protocols varies by region and State. Medical direction can also be administered online, or direction provided via electronic telecommunications to onscene or in-transit EMS personnel. By convention, online medical direction is immediately available and provided by a physician at a medical facility designated by the EMS agency.

To attempt to describe these agency components and relationships, a football analogy may be helpful. Protocols are to the EMS providers as the playbook is to the players. The medical director is the head coach for the entire team. As the protocols are put into play, there may be times the quarterback needs to quickly confer with the coach or assistant coach about a specific play in the field, and that is done using a radio in the same manner EMS providers use online medical direction.

EMS Agency Design Types

Today, virtually all communities throughout the United States have some type of EMS system. Though community expectations for an EMS system may vary based on locale and a particular community's risk tolerance levels, most modern EMS systems were designed by State statute and by local agency leaders to address the communities' need for a provision of timely, skilled emergency care at the point of illness or injury. EMS systems vary in clinical sophistication, performance measures, and economic efficiency.[12] There are different configurations of EMS systems in the United States and there is minimal evidence and considerable debate as to which approach may be the most effective.

Nearly all Americans have access to the 9-1-1 emergency phone number. This is the entry point into an EMS system that most people use. In some areas, trained call-takers and dispatchers use structured emergency medical dispatch programs to perform call triage, dispatch the most appropriate response personnel, and provide prearrival instructions to bystanders so that basic care can begin prior to EMS arriving. While the use of emergency medical dispatch programs is not consistent across the United States, their implementation and use is ever-increasing.

How emergency response resources are deployed following dispatch to calls for assistance is dependent upon a community's system configuration. In many communities, first responders are deployed from municipal fire or police departments. Ambulances (transport units) may also be deployed from fire departments, hospitals, third service, or private provider locations. Volunteer fire and rescue agencies were an early and common provider of both first responder and ambulance transport services, and remain an integral part of many EMS systems.

There are at least two EMS provider levels in most communities. These include basic life support (BLS) and ALS providers. Generally, BLS response units will have equipment sufficient to address initial patient care intervention including oxygen, fundamental airway support devices, bandaging and splinting devices, as well as automated external defibrillators (AEDs). ALS response units will have more highly trained and certified EMS providers and carry all the BLS equipment, in addition to complex patient intervention equipment such as advanced airway devices, intravenous fluids, medications, and cardiac monitors typically capable of 12-lead electrocardiography, transcutaneous pacing, as well as defibrillators capable of defibrillation and synchronized cardioversion.

Some EMS agencies may not be responsible for initial 9-1-1 responses. These agencies may be needed in special circumstances such as supplemental transport services (e.g., aeromedical units, critical or neonatal care units, etc.) or interfacility transport needs. Based on the agency configuration, they may offer BLS, ALS, or both levels of care.

Listed below are brief descriptions of the most common agency types in the United States. It is important to note the following descriptions are generic in nature; there are exceptions to these descriptions and one agency may fit into multiple categories.

Multiple-Role EMS Agency

A multiple-role EMS agency will cross-train their personnel to provide various services. A common example of a multiple-role EMS agency is a fire-based EMS agency. There are also multiple-role EMS agencies which provide rescue services, but not fire suppression. Less common are combined public safety agencies that provide cross-trained personnel to provide all three services of law enforcement, fire, and EMS services.

In fire-based EMS agencies, medical responses are provided by fire department personnel trained as emergency responders, EMTs, or paramedics. The integration of EMS into the public safety sector makes use of preexisting transportation infrastructure and personnel who are already trained to function in emergency conditions.

Single-Role EMS Agency

A single-role EMS agency provides EMS services only and personnel are not cross-trained to provide firefighting or other additional services. Single-role EMS agencies may be municipality based or privately owned and work closely and cooperatively with other public safety agencies.

Hospital-Based EMS Transport Agency

A hospital-based EMS agency, in the simplest of terms, means that a hospital has oversight and operational responsibility of an EMS agency. These types of agencies may be public or private and vary in how their EMS care is deployed. Some hospital-based agencies may operate in combination with the other community emergency responders (e.g., fire department) while others may provide a separate and independent EMS agency. Traditionally, hospital-based agencies are private and may be either for-profit or not-for-profit entities. These types of agencies are often found connected with large teaching hospitals and their provider base may also function within other areas of the hospital at times.

Private EMS Agency

Private EMS agencies are individually or corporately owned and operated companies. These agencies may provide nonemergent or emergent ambulance transport services. In the nonemergent setting, private EMS agencies often provide extensive scheduled intrafacility services to a community or region. Private EMS agencies can be for-profit or not-for-profit.

Third-Service EMS Agency

In a third-service EMS agency, there is an entity that provides EMS service in a manner that is separate but alongside the fire and police public safety personnel in the community. For example, a community may have the fire department provide the first response to initiate immediate patient care which will be followed by the arrival of a separate governmental-based EMS agency or a private EMS service to provide the ambulance transports.

Public Utility EMS Agency

In a public utility EMS agency structure, the local government regulates, oversees, and coordinates the provision of EMS throughout the community. The government is responsible for the entire agency performance and may own the equipment, apparatus, and perform insurance billing, but will contract with a separate entity for the personnel requirements.

EMS Agency Staffing Types

Teamwork is an integral component of successful EMS delivery and the medical director needs to understand how an agency's culture, procedures, protocols, and State regulations affect the service delivery. The backbone of any EMS agency is its personnel. Agency types vary from community to community based on a number of factors that include agency history and evolution, funding resources, geographic and population densities, as well as community risk tolerances and expectations. EMS agencies may be made up entirely of career (paid) personnel, volunteers, or a combination of the two. A medical director will interact with the administrative, operational, and provider level personnel of an agency. This interaction requires skills to perform as an educator, an advisor, a coach, a mentor, a leader, and a technical expert.

Career

EMS agencies that are career-based pay their providers for performing their role as an EMS provider. In general, EMS agencies in urban areas typically have career personnel. Within these areas, there is a strong trend for the municipal fire department to provide both EMS and fire suppression services, either as a single or multirole provider format. Other urban delivery models include those where single-role EMS personnel are employed by a municipality, hospital, or with private ambulance companies.[13]

Career-based EMS agencies can achieve a great deal of standardization and consistency of staffing levels as agency leaders can manage the workforce through employer oversight and mandated activities.

Volunteer

Volunteer EMS agencies rely on personnel who participate with the service without typically being compensated for their time. While some urban agencies have active involvement from volunteer EMS providers, the majority of volunteer-based EMS agencies are located in suburban and rural settings. The amount of volunteer activity within the EMS industry makes it unique when compared to other types of health-care occupations.

Volunteer-based EMS agencies may experience more variability in their staffing level consistency and face challenges in managing a force that is confronted with competing time commitments and increasing demands of training and continuing education requirements, particularly at the ALS certification levels.

Combination

A combination agency will use both career and volunteer personnel. Combination agencies attempt to achieve some cost savings by using volunteers, thereby reducing the amount of salaried employees. However, the viability of a combination agency is strongly dependent on the community's ability to supply and sustain a pool of interested and engaged volunteers.

Medical directors may find that many agencies experience an evolutionary process where the agency may be transitioning from a complete volunteer agency to a combination agency, and then into a full career agency. Regardless of the EMS agency type, all providers must be held to the same standard of patient care excellence.

The delivery of EMS can be physically and mentally demanding, and dangerous situations and environments are frequently encountered. Occupational injury rates are common and EMS personnel experience occupational death rates comparable to firefighters and police officers.[14] EMS agencies may experience EMS provider turnover due to injury, burnout, or occupational-related stress and a medical director must understand how the environment can have significant impacts on the providers.

Types of Response Service

EMS agencies develop and are designed to meet a community's needs and expectations. In an effort to match responding resources with the need, agencies may offer only one service level response and transport or be tiered to offer both BLS and ALS services.

As a medical director, it is critical that you become familiar with all the organizations involved with the EMS agency in your area and understand how these entities contribute to the structure and design of that agency.

Single-Tier Response Service

In a single-tier agency design, every EMS response, regardless of call type, receives the same level of personnel expertise and equipment allocation. These agencies provide initial response and transport at one level of care, which may be all BLS or all ALS.

Tiered Response Service

In a tiered agency delivery design, levels of response are broken down into layers or tiers. An example of this type of service is to have first responders provide the BLS tier and then have paramedic-staffed ambulances provide the ALS tier of service. Tiered agencies will often use various vehicle types in their service delivery model (e.g., first response sedans or sport utility vehicles (SUVs), fire apparatus, as well as ambulances, etc.).

In a tiered agency, the initial call triage performed by 9-1-1 call-taker becomes a key element in matching the resources dispatched to the caller's needs.

Resource Deployment

In addition to whether an agency has a tiered approach to service delivery, deployment of resources is another consideration in agency design. There are typically two types of resource deployment: fixed or dynamic.

Fixed Deployment

In a fixed deployment model, EMS response vehicles are dispatched from a static location within a response area, like a fire or EMS station that is strategically positioned within the community for efficient response.

Dynamic Deployment

Dynamic deployment is often referred to as **system status management**. In this deployment model, EMS response vehicles are positioned at various locations within a given response area. These posting sites are selected following a retrospective analysis of call volume and locations in order to statistically predict where the next call may occur. Vehicles may post in parking lots, buildings, or park along a street location and their positions may change based on real-time factors influencing the system.

Emergency Medical Dispatch

As previously mentioned, nearly all Americans can access 9-1-1 as the entry point to access the services of an EMS system. Municipally-operated 9-1-1 communications centers are referred to as Public Safety Answering Points (PSAPs). PSAPs are commonly a fire or rescue, law enforcement, or jointly controlled and operated center. Depending on the municipality, private EMS agencies may not be included in the 9-1-1 deployment resources, unless they are specifically contracted to provide a service to the municipality.

PSAPs can differ in design and resources. Some PSAPs are cross functional managing all calls for public safety resources (EMS, fire, or police) and personnel are cross-trained in the call-taking process, emergency medical dispatch (EMD) procedures and dispatch of resources. Other PSAPs may be segregated into separate sections. As an example, the 9-1-1 call may be answered by a police trained call-taker who will quickly determine the nature of the call as EMS, fire, or police. If the call is medical in nature, the police call-taker would forward it to the EMS section of the PSAP for subsequent questioning and dispatch of resources.

Regardless of how the PSAP is designed or 9-1-1 calls are routed, there are common fundamental activities. EMD programs should employ a system of medical questioning to assess the caller's actual emergency, gain additional information, and/or offer basic medical care intervention instructions over the telephone, called "prearrival instructions" (e.g., bleeding control, cardiopulmonary resuscitation (CPR)). EMD programs use a finite list of common chief complaints, each having associated predetermined questions. Answers to these questions ultimately dictate the resources sent to the scene and how those resources will travel (nonemergency driving or use of lights and sirens). There are several commercially available EMD programs for which the agency's medical director working with the PSAP manager could adopt for use.

Traditionally, the medical director had oversight responsibilities for providers in direct contact with patients. With the evolving standard of care for EMD, many medical directors now have program oversight duties in their agency's PSAP. To provide appropriate EMD program oversight, the medical director must develop a working knowledge of the following related items:

• scope of practice for EMD programs;

• any local, State, and national level legislation related to 9-1-1 PSAP functions;

• the PSAP's general operations, organizational structure, administration, training, and quality improvement activities; and

• the authority of the medical director relating to developing, approving, revising dispatch procedures and protocols, and their role in overall quality management of the PSAP.

Of critical importance, the medical director must ensure there is seamless transition between the EMD program's protocols and prearrival instructions and the EMS agency's field response protocols and policies.

Emergency Response Components

Local emergency response agencies often provide an "all-hazards" response capability. This means the agency's resources will respond to any and all types of natural or manmade incidents. During large scale or technically complex incidents, the EMS resources need to function in a collaborative manner with other response agencies. An incident management system is an organizational structure that integrates resources in a hierarchal organization to improve coordination, effectiveness, and efficiency in the management of an event.

The National Incident Management System (NIMS) is used in the United States for the coordination of Federal, State, and local agencies. The Federal Emergency Management Agency (FEMA) has well-developed training programs in NIMS. The level of the training program required is based on the level of responsibility an individual is expected to have during an incident. Regardless of the type, scope, or scale of an incident, a medical director must become trained and operationally familiar with NIMS.

All medical directors should complete FEMA IS-100.b: *Introduction to Incident Command System (ICS)*, FEMA IS-200.b: *ICS for Single Resources and Initial Action Incidents*, and FEMA IS-700.a: *NIMS An Introduction*. Depending on the local community's threat assessment, the EMS agency may want the medical director to complete additional NIMS training such as FEMA IS-230b: *Fundamentals of Emergency Management*, FEMA ICS-300: *Intermediate ICS for Expanding Incidents for Operational First Responders*, FEMA IS-346: *An Orientation to Hazardous Materials for Medical Personnel*, FEMA IS-520: *Introduction to Continuity of Operations Planning for Pandemic Influenzas*, and FEMA IS-800.b: *National Response Framework, An Introduction*. The medical director should work closely with their local agency to identify the appropriate classes. FEMA's website has a wealth of information explaining NIMS training and links to online courses. The link for more information is: www.fema.gov/emergency/nims/

Medical directors must have a comprehensive understanding of their EMS agency's role and responsibility before, during, and following incident response, stabilization, and resolution. The medical director is responsible for being engaged in planning, overseeing patient care, performing agency improvement activities, and having knowledge of related peer-reviewed medical literature, as well as industry standards, so that future incidents have better outcomes, increased efficiency, and enhanced effectiveness.

In some EMS agencies, providers may operate in difficult conditions, remote areas, or need to perform specialized skills. Oversight of these unique environments that require specialized skills and training will require specialized medical direction. The frequency with which an EMS agency engages in these events will influence the amount of specific knowledge and involvement a medical director will need to have.

Listed below is an overview of several response components that may be applicable to a medical director's individual agency in their all-hazard environment.

Disasters or Multiple and Mass Casualty Incidents

EMS agencies will respond to disasters of all types and scales. Disaster planning is vital and often complex in nature. A medical director should become engaged in the planning process and understand what the agency's expected response will be. A local resource that a medical director may find extremely helpful is the agency's emergency management division or a community-based organization responsible for local disaster response plans such as a Local Emergency Planning Committee (LEPC) or Emergency Management Agency (EMA).

The acronym MCI is typically used interchangeably when referring to both multiple and mass casualty incidents. Multiple casualty incidents are incidents involving multiple patients that can typically be managed using a system's existing resources. Multiple casualty incidents usually have an intense but relatively short operational period. In contrast, mass casualty incidents involve a greater number of patients and will overwhelm the responding agency or system's resources. Mass casualty incidents tend to have a greater, sustained period of operations. Multiple casualty incidents occur more often than mass casualty incidents or large scale disasters. In some busy urban areas, multiple casualty incidents may occur on a daily basis (e.g., crashes involving multiple vehicles and multiple patients).

Following the declaration of a MCI or a disaster, the incident management system will engage and a well-structured flow of incident control activities that include patient triage, treatment, and transportation should occur. A medical director should be familiar and involved with the agency's policies regarding the management of these incidents.

The National Fire Protection Association (NFPA) has a published industry standard related to disaster and MCI responses which the medical director may want to become familiar with. This is NFPA 1600, *Standard on Disaster/Emergency Management and Business Continuity Programs*.

Disasters and MCIs are situations where a medical director may be called to the scene by EMS personnel. Onscene roles and activities will be discussed later in the handbook.

Technical Rescue or Medical Search and Rescue

EMS resources may be called upon to provide medical support or be directly involved in technical rescue operations or search and rescue incidents. Technical rescues may include rope rescue, trench rescue, confined space rescue, swift water rescue, urban search and rescue, building collapses, or other specialized situations requiring a specific skill set. Personnel involved in these types of events are highly trained and deployed when conventional rescue techniques will not meet the needs of the specific incident.

Search and rescue incidents include the systematic search for persons who are lost or in distress on land or inland waterways. These incidents may occur in wilderness zones and include ski, cave, forest, and waterway areas.

Medical directors of these types of agencies must become familiar with the specific training requirements and nature of technical rescue incidents; although, all medical directors should be aware these could impact their local EMS resources. FEMA has designated Urban Search and Rescue (US&R) teams across the nation. US&R teams may have their own medical doctors who have received specialized training for the types of environments and responses these teams become activated for.

NFPA has a published industry standard related to technical rescue responses that the medical director may want to become familiar with. This publication is NFPA 1670, *Standard on Operations and Training for Technical Search and Rescue Incidents*.

Occupational Safety and Health Administration (OSHA) also has related industry standards that impact technical rescue operations. OSHA's regulation 29 CFR Part 1910: *Occupational Safety and Health Standards* has several subparts that medical directors should become familiar with.

Special or Mass Gatherings Events

Organizers of special events may seek preapproval for use of EMS agency resources to provide medical support for mass gathering events. Examples of mass gathering events can be sporting events, entertainment gatherings, rallies, and community activities. Preplanning activities are especially vital for these events and will require preevent analysis, staffing resource evaluation, and interagency coordination needs. Medical directors should be involved during the planning activities to understand the scope and demands that may be placed on the agency.

Hazardous Materials

A hazardous material (hazmat) is a substance or material that poses a risk to health, safety, or property and is governed by Federal regulations when transported in commerce. EMS agencies can be tasked with responding to a hazmat scene. All medical directors need to have a general knowledge of the medical issues involved in hazmat responses. Those medical directors who oversee hazmat teams must have additional training to be prepared for these types of incidents. There are some agencies with hazmat teams that are electing to implement programs, such as the Tox-Medic© program, for specialized advanced hazmat life support training, with a focus on chemical behavior and toxicology for paramedics that will provide medical surveillance and care to hazmat team members and patients exposed to chemical, biological, and nuclear exposure incidents.

NFPA has published industry standards related to hazmat emergency response which the medical director may want to become familiar with. Three hazmat-related NFPA standards are:

- NFPA 471, *Recommended Practice for Responding to Hazardous Materials Incidents.*

- NFPA 472, *Standard for Competence of Responders to Hazardous Materials/Weapons of Mass Destruction Incidents.*

- NFPA 473, *Standard for Competencies for EMS Personnel Responding to Hazardous Materials/Weapons of Mass Destruction Incidents.*

NFPA also has several standards related to provider protective ensembles to be worn during hazmat-related incidents that can be referenced if the medical director is requested to provide input on protective clothing for hazmat incidents.

OSHA's regulation 29 CFR Part 1910.120 and several subparts are applicable in these situations. In addition, the National Institute for Occupational Safety and Health (NIOSH) has publications related to the selection and wearing of respirators which are also applicable.

Wildland

Wildland refers to wilderness areas that are found in preserves, estates, farms, conservation preserves, ranches, national forests, national parks, and along rivers, gulches, or otherwise undeveloped areas within or near large urban areas. EMS providers may be called to support a wildland fire incident. Wildland incidents are typically based out of remote camp locations where providers from multiple areas will work together to render aid as needed.

A challenge in large scale wildland fire events is how responding EMS providers are covered by medical director oversight. An EMS provider's ability to function under the authority of their local medical director becomes questionable when responding into another State or on Federal property. If a medical director is involved with an agency that may provide wildland fire support, the medical director must become familiar with local, State, and Federal regulations regarding issues related to EMS provider physician oversight and protocol usage and consult with the local fire chief or emergency manager.

NFPA has a published industry standard related to wildland responses which the medical director may want to become familiar with. This is NFPA 1143, *Standard for Wildland Fire Management* and NFPA 1051, *Standard for Wildland Fire Fighter Professional Qualifications*. Other resources may be referenced from the National Wildfire Coordinating Group (NWCG), an organization with representatives from each Federal land management agencies and the National Association of State Foresters.

Tactical EMS

EMS providers may be requested to support high hazard tactical law enforcement incidents. In order to properly support these situations, there is specialized training available for tactical medics. Counter Narcotics and Terrorism Operational Medical Support (CONTOMS) is a nationally recognized tactical medical support program for law enforcement and military operations established by the HHS, DHS, and the U.S. Park Police.

CONTOMS offers a medical director's course that is specifically designed for those who will be providing medical direction for EMS providers operating in this type of role. Tactical environments require different approaches and procedures than the routine civilian emergency environment and this course outlines specific policies, protocols, and issues associated with overseeing a program of this nature.

Other organizations may also have tactical EMS-related training programs. As an example, the National Tactical Officers Association offers EMS provider tactical training and a specific medical director course is under development at this time.

Becoming a Medical Director

Physicians interested in becoming a medical director enter into an aspect of emergency medical care that is distinct from the emergency department. It will present a realm of challenges that will require analytical, clinical, managerial, and leadership skills. Medical direction is essential to ensure patient care that is high quality, efficient, effective, and safe for patients as well as for providers.

The handbook is designed for all agency medical directors--from small agencies and neophyte medical directors getting their initial field exposure through emergency medical services (EMS) ride-alongs, to medical directors in large systems with high-incident volume and a large staff where the medical director may be an integral part of administrative and field operations on a daily basis.

Role and Purpose of the Medical Director

The American College of Emergency Physicians (ACEP) highlighted the medical director as an integral component of the EMS agency, stating that the medical director should have ultimate authority over all clinical and patient care aspects of the EMS agency, with the specific job description dictated by local needs, including the authorization to "limit immediately the patient care activities of those who deviate from established standards or do not meet training standards."[15] EMS medical direction involves granting authorities to act and accepting responsibility for the delivery of EMS patient care. Medical direction is narrower than oversight in that it defines what treatments EMS providers render when presented with medical conditions. Medical oversight ensures that the care is rendered by competent medical professionals, consistent with accepted standards. Medical oversight and direction are essential to all EMS systems as they help to ensure the appropriate delivery of emergency medical care to those with medical needs. The Federal Interagency Committee on EMS (FICEMS), as well as the National Association of Emergency Medical Technicians (NAEMT), stressed the importance of medical oversight in every EMS system; equally important in day-to-day EMS operations as during catastrophic events.

Across the United States, EMS providers obtain certification or licensure through a department or office located within their State government structure. However, in many States, this certification or licensure does not give permission for the EMS provider to function without being under the supervision of a licensed EMS agency and medical director. The medical director is responsible to ensure the patient care activities performed by EMS providers are appropriate, within their scope of practice, and within operational expectations. While advanced life support (ALS) agencies must have a medical director for paramedics to perform advanced therapies and patient care interventions, there is variability among State requirements for a medical director to oversee the basic life support (BLS) providers in an agency. Medical directors need to check with their State EMS office to determine what requirements are specified.

EMS providers function under the supervision of a medical director for patient care-related activities and the providers are dually accountable to their agency's hierarchical structure. It is critical that the medical director work collaboratively with the agency's leaders to ensure the EMS program administrative, operational, and clinical components are cohesive and complementary. The medical director and EMS agency's leadership must forge a positive, constructive, and collaborative relationship to enable the agency to be an effective and productive organization.

Scope of Responsibility

Agency Oversight

The medical director will be responsible for the general patient care-related activities of a particular agency. There are many facets of an EMS agency in which a medical director should be engaged in including education and training activities, protocol and policy development, quality improvement activities, liaison, and corrective actions related to patient care actions by providers. Ideally, the medical director should have a strong familiarity with all the EMS providers within their agency. Additional and specific agency-level activities will be discussed in further detail in subsequent chapters of this handbook.

Education and Training of the Medical Director

A medical director's specific qualifications, responsibilities, and authority differ across States and among individual EMS agencies. There are several consensus standard agencies and professional associations that have identified the professional education and training requirements for the medical director position.

Postgraduate Education

Physicians who complete a residency in emergency medicine are exposed to the fundamentals of EMS systems as part of their core education. For well over a decade, fellowships in EMS have been available to interested residency graduates who have a special interest in out-of-hospital patient care.

In September 2010, the American Board of Emergency Medicine (ABEM) announced the creation of an EMS subspecialty for physicians. This announcement followed years of focused efforts by EMS stakeholders such as the National Association of EMS Physicians (NAEMSP), ACEP, ABEM, and the Society for Academic Emergency Medicine. ABEM expects to begin the examination process in 2013. For eligibility requirements and additional information, the following website can be accessed: www.abem.org/PUBLIC/portal/alias_Rainbow/lang_en-US/tabID_4128/DesktopDefault.aspx

With the advent of the EMS subspecialty, EMS fellowship training programs will become fully accredited by the Accreditation Council for Graduate Medical Education (ACGME). Additional fellowship information can be accessed at the ABEM website specified above or at the NAEMSP website: www.naemsp.org/fellowshipprograms.html

State Requirements

A physician seeking endorsement as an EMS medical director must hold a current, unrestricted license to practice medicine or osteopathy issued by their State's Board of Medicine. States typically require a physician to complete a medical director training course. Many States have developed their own training course and many accept completion of a nationally recognized course.

Initial medical director training may be available at the local, regional, and State level. Many medical directors will elect to attend an initial training course at national conferences such as NAEMSP's offerings. In addition to attending an onsite class, there are online courses, such as the Critical Illness and Trauma Foundation (CITF) offering. CITF offers an online medical director training course which is based on National Highway Traffic Safety Administration (NHTSA), ACEP, and the NAEMSP guidelines for preparing medical directors. States may enter into a contract with CITF to support this training for that State's agency medical directors. If a particular State does not have a contractual agreement with CITF, individual physicians can register for the course for a fee. The CITF online course can be accessed by the following link: www.medicaldirectoronline.org

In many States, if the physician is Board Certified in Emergency Medicine (by the ABEM or the American Board of Osteopathic Emergency Medicine (AOBEM)), there may only be a requirement to complete the State's medical director training program. If the medical director is not Board Certified in Emergency Medicine, then many States require current certification in Advanced Cardiac Life Support (ACLS), Advanced Trauma Life Support (ATLS), and Pediatric Advanced Life Support (PALS) in addition to the successful completion of the State's medical director training course. However, there are variations in what States require for their initial medical director training, as well as the continuing education requirements. Physicians should contact their State EMS office for assistance in locating class offerings. Specific requirements for your State may also be found by following the link below to your State EMS agency: www.nesemso.org/About/StateEMSAgencies/StateEMSagencyListing.asp

Consensus Standards and Professional Associations

Numerous consensus positions or standards can be found addressing the initial and continuing education of a medical director. Though many medical directors are not Board Certified in Emergency Medicine, ACEP, NAEMSP, National Association of State EMS Officials (NASEMSO), and some States encourage the medical director to be Board Certified in Emergency Medicine. All of these organizations have position descriptions, educational materials, and other supporting materials that can be accessed on their websites which aid in the education of a prospective, new, or incumbent medical director. Links to these organizations are

> ACEP: www.acep.org
>
> NAEMSP: www.naemsp.org
>
> NASEMSO: www.nasemso.org

An Institute of Medicine (IOM) report titled "Emergency Medical Services at the Crossroads" released in June 2006 highlighted the need for stronger leadership within the EMS agency in order to make it more effective. EMS fellowship opportunities exist to help prepare interested physicians with the knowledge and leadership skills that are needed to become an effective medical director.

In general, the various EMS industry standards and guidelines contain commonalities when identifying qualifications for a medical director. These qualifications and skills can be summarized as:

- licensed to practice medicine or osteopathy (M.D. or D.O.);

- Board Certified or Board-prepared in Emergency Medicine (not required in many circumstances, but preferred);

- clinically active in emergency medicine;

- understanding of the design and operation of EMS agencies;

- familiar with local/regional EMS activity;

- familiar with administrative and legislative process that impact EMS;

- familiar with the scope of EMS skills (BLS and ALS) and communications systems;

- understanding of emergency medical dispatch (EMD) principles and processes;

- familiar with providing online and offline medical direction activities;

- involvement with training of EMS providers;

- involvement with quality improvement activities in all aspects of EMS delivery; and

- knowledge of local, regional, and State mass casualty and disaster plans.

Agency Training

Once the physician assumes the medical director role for the EMS agency, the agency needs to provide support and specific training for the new medical director. The agency should provide an orientation so the new medical director can be introduced to all personnel and understand the organization's structure and operations. The orientation should include a tour of all facilities and orientation to apparatus and equipment typically used.

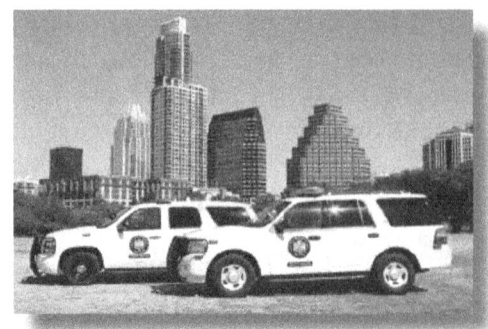

If the medical director is expected to operate any of the agency's vehicles, then the agency needs to ensure the medical director receives Emergency Vehicle Operator Course (EVOC) training or equivalent courses approved by the agency's State EMS office.

As required by Occupational Safety and Health Administration (OSHA) (29 CFR Part 1910.1030), the medical director will also need agency provided infection control training prior to performing any field exposures or ride-alongs with agency personnel.

If the agency provides any specialized response components such as those discussed in the previous chapter, there may be additional and specialized training the medical director needs to obtain.

The agency needs to provide copies of, and educate the medical director on existing standard operating procedures (SOPs), training curriculums, and protocols.

Continuing Education for the Medical Director

The continuing education requirement for a medical director will also vary from State to State. Some States will require an annual or biannual update for medical directors to ensure their knowledge base is maintained regarding State regulations and to discuss emerging industry trends or hot topics. If not specifically required by the State, many EMS agencies will prefer if their medical director is not Board Certified in Emergency Medicine, that they maintain specific certifications such as ACLS, ATLS, PALS, as well as satisfying the educational requirements for the physician's primary board certification.

In addition to the NAEMSP (whose annual conference is dedicated to topics related to EMS medical directors), there are numerous professional organizations with EMS sections that sponsor national conferences. These offer continuing education relevant to a medical director's role. These events not only provide needed continuing education credits, they expose the medical director to networking opportunities with other medical directors and industry professionals.

Regardless of State regulation or agency requirement, a dedicated medical director will pursue ongoing educational activities, exposure to the out-of-hospital environment, and contact with providers they oversee.

Affiliation Agreements

When a physician decides to act as a medical director, a written agreement with the agency is needed and may be required by State rules or statues. This written agreement needs to provide a position description, the expected tasks, performance criteria, agreed upon compensation, provided resources, liability coverage, and the process for dispute resolution.

Agency, municipal, and State regulations will assist in defining the medical director role and authority. The medical director's scope of responsibility and authority must be clearly delineated in the position description and written agreement with both the agency and medical director educated on all topics within the agreement.

The form of affiliation agreement can vary from agency to agency. The medical director must understand the ramifications of the written agreement and the advantages and/or disadvantages of the form of the relationship. For example, if the medical director becomes an employee of the agency, there may be perceived advantages such as benefit coverage (e.g., insurance, etc.) or automatic tax-related deductions that may not be included in a contract form of agreement. However, there may also be perceived disadvantages by having the medical director in an employee status that is accountable to an agency supervisor or potential restrictions on lobbying activities that may not be present in a memorandum of agreement (MOA).

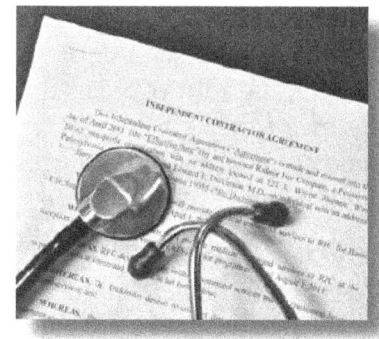

The medical director must carefully assess all factors when considering and negotiating the type and content of the agreement. Regardless of the type of agreement, a part of any negotiation is the need for the agency to support the medical director. The agency should provide support to the medical director in the form of resources and training. Examples include administrative support, providing training for agency-specific requirements, access to facilities and personnel, financial support for conference attendance, or other continuing education needs.

To fully understand the differences between the forms of affiliation agreements, the medical director should seek independent legal and tax professional consultation prior to entering into any agreement to ensure adequate protection and that expectations are clearly defined. This action should be taken regardless of if the position is uncompensated or compensated in nature. Employed physicians also need to discuss these relationships with their employer, as there may be both contract and liability issues. The handbook contains a sample affiliation agreement in the appendix.

Hire/Employee

In some cases, the medical director will be a competitively hired or appointed position within the agency. With this type of arrangement, the position of the medical director becomes an employee of the agency which may be either an appointed, part-time or full-time position dependent on the size, complexity, scope, and needs of the agency.

Independent Contractor

Agencies may advertise a request for proposal or invitation to bid where they will contract for medical direction services with the selected party. Simply stated, a contract is a legally binding agreement between the parties and the agreement is governed by contract law. There are general requirements typically found in contracts which include the contract purpose, the legal issues associated with the contract, identification of the parties represented by the contract, an offer and acceptance to perform the requested services, what resources are agreed upon, responsibilities, penalties, and the process to terminate the contract. Contracts can cover either uncompensated or compensated relationships.

Memorandum of Understanding and Memorandum of Agreements

Agencies may also enter into a memorandum of understanding (MOU) or an MOA with the medical director and may also address uncompensated or compensated arrangements.

MOUs typically define and clarify the relationship between two parties. One major difference between a contract and an MOU is that the MOU is usually not entirely binding on the parties. Medical directors may feel uncomfortable with this type of agreement, especially in the areas of potential legal representation and liability coverage.

Similarly, an MOA is a promise between parties to cooperatively work together on an agreed upon project. The MOA can establish the expectations of how the parties will pursue a positive, cooperative effort. There is typically a list of terms that may be binding on how the parties will work cohesively together within the terms of the agreement. Once again, medical directors may believe an MOA will not be comprehensive enough if a legal issue was to arise during the course of the relationship.

Performance Expectations

While the medical director's position description will identify the duties and responsibilities, it does not identify how the medical director will perform them. Performance expectations are the measurement tool for understanding if the duties and responsibilities are being met. The EMS agency's administration should clearly communicate the medical director's performance expectations. It is critical for both the agency and the medical director to understand and ensure that a balance is achieved between the performance expectations and time commitments.

Performance expectations are to be specific, measurable, realistically achievable, results-or outcomes-oriented, and have associated time lines where appropriate. This information is often included in the position's job description, contract, MOU, or MOA content. Examples of how a medical director's identified responsibility can be further defined by performance expectations are as follows:

Example 1:

Responsibility: The medical director shall serve on local, regional, and national committees and/or boards as mutually agreed upon by the agency's leadership and the medical director.

Performance Expectations

1. The medical director shall attend a minimum of 75 percent of local EMS committee meetings. Meetings will be held the second Thursday of each month unless otherwise specified.

2. The medical director will chair the Continuous Quality Improvement Committee. Meetings are to be held quarterly.

3. The medical director shall attend a minimum of 50 percent of regional EMS council meetings.

Example 2:

Responsibility: The agency agrees to provide needed resources and benefits to the medical director as mutually agreed upon by the agency's leadership and the medical director.

Performance Expectations

1. The agency will provide up to three periodical subscriptions as identified by the medical director directly related to the medical director's position and responsibilities.

2. The agency will provide financial support for the medical director to attend one regional, State, or national level conference on an annual basis. Costs of financial support will not exceed $1,500 per annual occurrence.

3. The agency will provide two work uniforms and one set of personal protective gear to be worn during emergency incident responses or field-related activities.

4. The agency will provide administrative support for correspondence proofreading and formatting, copying of documents, and filing support for materials directly related to the medical director's position and responsibilities.

5.   If onscene medical director support is requested, the agency will provide a driver and arrange for pick up or rendezvous point with the medical director to be transported to the scene in an official vehicle.

Compensation and Benefits

Dependent on the size and scope of the EMS agency with whom the medical director will be involved, the agreement to serve as a medical director may or may not include compensation and/or benefits. The EMS agency has an obligation to support the medical director and provide the appropriate resources in the form of agreed upon compensation (hourly or salaried), materials and personnel assets (costs associated with uniform, equipment, travel, continuing education, or professional organization memberships, etc.), and liability protections. However, an EMS agency's resources will vary depending on locale, and many will require charitable contribution of the medical director's time and expertise. It is critical that an EMS medical director ensure personal protection for both liability and injury, despite the lack of resources available to the EMS agency.

Workers' Compensation

Each State identifies and controls the workers' compensation insurance policies. This coverage is mandatory for employers and covers their employees for any injuries they incur in the course and scope of their employment.

If a medical director has an employee/employer relationship with their agency, workers' compensation may be a recognized benefit afforded to the medical director. However, if the medical director has a contractual MOU or MOA for their services, workers' compensation coverage is almost never included.

Dependent upon the situation and service agreement, an EMS agency may require the medical director to obtain their own workers' compensation insurance for the medical director and any other staff that the medical director may employ. The agency may also require proof of such coverage or proof that workers' compensation is not required by law. Agencies may also require the medical director to indemnify and hold the agency harmless from any and all claims for these obligations.

Medical directors need to check with their agency's leadership for specific workers' compensation requirements and understand how the relationship may be impacted by the form of agreed upon affiliation agreement.

Continuing Education

If an EMS agency requires their medical director to maintain specific certifications or perform certain continuing education activities, the agency may bear some of the obligation to support the medical director in the activity. For example, if the agency requires the medical director to perform field work, then the specific initial and ongoing training to properly prepare the medical director (e.g., infection control, emergency vehicle operator course, communication device use) should be provided by the agency.

The expectation for this arrangement must be clearly stated in the job description, contract, MOU, or MOA. Often, professional journal subscriptions or conference attendance are a negotiated benefit.

IRS Requirements

Unless the medical director is an employee of the agency, the medical director will be individually responsible for all Federal and State taxes. This responsibility will include Social Security, Medicare taxes, and self-employment-related taxes and obligations including Federal and State income tax withholding, Social Security contributions, and similar obligations related to the medical director's independent contract, MOU, or MOA. As with the workers' compensation issue, the agency may require the medical director to indemnify and hold the agency harmless from any and all claims for these obligations.

The medical director should consult an independent tax professional for further review and guidance.

Dissolution

When the relationship between the medical director and the EMS agency is no longer going to continue, a dissolution or termination of the service agreement needs to occur.

Typically, any form of agreement to serve should contain language of how the agreement would be terminated. A critical component in this area would be the timing of the intent to terminate notification on either party's behalf. Typically, agencies will require a minimum of 90-days notice so that a replacement medical director can be obtained without experiencing a disruption in service delivery. Other critical components for a medical director to consider with this issue is how property owned by the agency is returned, how compensation is adjusted or reconciled, and how liability protection is addressed for any future cases that develop, which relate back to the time covered by the medical director's activity.

Liability Coverage

Although many physicians have malpractice insurance coverage that may extend to some of the activities of medical director, they are unlikely to have coverage for all potential liabilities associated with the medical director position, role, and responsibilities. In fact, the medical director's typical professional liability coverage may have coverage gaps related to the associated EMS activities being performed.

The medical director must have a clear understanding of who, what, and when their activities are covered by the agency's liability policies. Just as important to knowing what activities are included in the liability coverage, the medical director must know what activities may be excluded from the coverage. In addition to medical malpractice coverage, medical directors need to carry errors and omission insurance, and be covered under the general liability policy of their agency. If the medical director is considered to be serving in a leadership role of the agency, then director's and officer's insurance coverage may also be needed.

Obtaining adequate liability coverage as a medical director can be challenging. Resources to obtain adequate coverage include the agency's insurance carrier, a rider to your clinical practice's insurance carrier, an independent insurance broker who deals in "unique" coverage circumstances (large, national/international broker), and insurance available through professional organizations. Medical directors should seek independent consultation with an attorney familiar with liability issues for additional guidance related to requirements for adequate coverage. This action should be taken regardless of if the position is uncompensated or compensated in nature.

It is recommended that a medical director establish a working relationship with the agency's risk management section. Medical directors must have a thorough understanding to ensure they have comprehensive liability protection either through the agency's self-insurance, indemnification, and/or separate insurance policy coverage. It cannot be stressed enough that the standard liability protection possessed by all practicing physicians will be inadequate to cover a physician for medical direction activities. In the appendix, there is a sample liability insurance form.

Medical Malpractice Coverage

Medical malpractice is an act of commission or omission by a health-care provider when their care deviates from accepted practice standards which results in a patient's injury or death. The professional liability policy must include medical malpractice coverage which is designed to cover risk and liabilities that occur in the field setting where patient care has been provided.

Errors and Omission Coverage

In general, errors and omission insurance helps provide coverage for defense costs and damage awards that may be associated with professional liability claims. Errors and omission coverage must cover the risk associated with any nonpatient care activities (e.g., oversight and training exposures) the medical director engages in. Errors and omission insurance typically does not provide coverage for intentional, fraudulent, or illegal activities, and many policies will not cover punitive damages.

General Liability Coverage

EMS agencies generally have a commercial general liability policy (in some States, this is a requirement to become licensed). A medical director requires some coverage that is found in general liability policies. If the medical director uses equipment or a vehicle owned by the EMS agency, the medical director must assume there could be risk associated with that equipment or vehicle. Usually, the owner would be liable for damages caused by the equipment, but additional coverage specifically for the medical director to use non-owned equipment or vehicles should be considered.

Issues related to employment practices are another large area of general liability exposure for the medical director. The EMS agency should consider obtaining Employment Practices Liability (EPL) coverage for these types of claims, and if the medical director is involved in employment-related activities or decision-making, the medical director could be included in this coverage.

Directors' and Officers' Coverage

Director and Officer insurance provides coverage against legal defense costs and indemnity for the agency, directors and officers, as well as personnel in legal claims that assert internal mismanagement or performance of wrongful acts while acting in director or officer capacity for the agency.

Indemnification

Medical directors need to require their EMS agency to include indemnification of the medical director in their service agreement. Indemnification simply means that the EMS agency will agree to assume the financial responsibility associated with defending the claim or lawsuit and will be responsible for monetary awards if an individual prevails in a lawsuit related to the performance of duties by the medical director. If there is not an indemnification clause in the agreement, the medical director could be held personally liable for the financial damages awarded in a prevailing lawsuit (subject, of course, to any applicable insurance coverage that might be in place).

Areas of Caution for Medical Directors

The medical director is recognized as a leader of an EMS agency, but the position is not the only leadership position in the agency. While the medical director is responsible for overseeing the clinical patient care components of the EMS agency, they must work in concert with the agency's administrative and operational leaders.

As with any position of organizational leadership, a medical director is expected to comply with accepted professional, moral, and ethical activities. The medical director must ensure their actions are performed in accordance with standard workplace practices and are carried out in a nondiscriminatory manner.

There are a few areas when the lines between clinical, administrative, and operational practice become blurred and seem to carry over into the different realms. As previously mentioned, the medical director supervises the EMS providers' medical practice. The medical director may withdraw their supervision of an EMS provider if the provider's performances of procedures or medical interventions are questioned. The provider's employer is generally responsible for the hiring, promoting, terminating, or other employment actions.

When faced with these situations, the agency's leaders must work closely together to ensure fair and equitable actions are taken without infringing on an individual's rights or taking action which may be deemed beyond the leader's scope of authority. Discussed below are some of the general areas that a medical director's scope of authority may be limited and direct involvement within should be approached with caution.

Hiring and Promotional Decisions

Depending on the agency, the medical director's involvement with hiring and advancement opportunities of the personnel may be limited. The EMS agency may request the medical director's involvement in the development of the criteria such as medical qualifications and credentialing, but the medical director should not participate in the actual hiring or promotion decision. Agencies may request the medical director review applications or resume information as it pertains to medical knowledge or credentialing, but actual decisions to hire or promote individuals will not likely be a decision that directly involves the medical director. However, if the medical director also functions as a managing partner of the agency (e.g., private- or hospital-based agency), the involvement in hiring and promotional decisions may more directly involve the medical director due to their dual agency role.

Provider Disciplinary Actions

The medical director is responsible for the clinical application of patient care policies, procedures, and protocols. When there are situations where individuals may not have performed as expected, the medical director may be involved in determining the circumstances and identifying appropriate remedial actions, but may not be further involved in decisions if disciplinary actions will take place. Often, such determinations and remediation involve collaborative investigations with administrative leaders in the EMS agency. There may be workplace regulations, identified in Federal, State, or local regulations that describe how the investigation is performed, including requirements for specific steps and notifications. The medical director should be knowledgeable of these due process requirements prior to the initiation of any investigative process.

There may be occurrences where the medical director may limit or revoke a member's privileges to provide patient care. Any further decisions related to the continued affiliation of the individual with the agency based on the provider's restriction from patient care environment are the responsibility of the agency's administration and/or State or local regulation. The medical director must recognize that agency-level disciplinary actions related to the direct employer-employee relationship are separate and the medical director should not become involved in those specific deliberations. As previously stated, if the medical director has a dual management role in the agency, there may be more participation in disciplinary issues beyond what is generally described above.

Budget and Procurement Regulations

Budget and procurement activities can be highly structured and governed by regulatory requirements. While the medical director may provide input and recommendations specific to patient care initiatives, the final decision, and regulatory compliance should be carried out by the agency's administrative and operational leaders.

The medical director may become engaged in advocating for budgetary needs with the appointed and political leaders associated with the EMS agency.

Conflict of Interest Considerations

A medical director is bound to maintain the highest ethical standards in the performance of their duties at all times. One of the areas where ethical issues can arise involves conflict of interests. The medical director should always maintain an awareness of potential professional, political, or financial conflicts of interest that may arise. In the event that a conflict of interest exists, it is crucial to ensure that your agency is made aware of this in writing. As a contractor, the medical director cannot be compelled to participate in a decision or action that they believe to be a conflict of interest.

Potential conflicts of interest include

- conflict between two separate EMS agencies, both of whom employ the same medical director;

- financial conflicts of interest if the medical director, or immediate family members, have stock, corporate holdings, royalty arrangements, etc., with products or services that might be used by the EMS agency;

- personal relationships with personnel for whom you oversee;

- conflict between the EMS agency and the hospital where the medical director is employed either directly or indirectly; and

- nepotism situations or concerns.

Steps for conflict resolution:

1. Disclose conflict to all parties.

2. Attempt to remediate the conflict of interest. Options may include

   a. If there is an assistant medical director, assign the decisionmaking activity to the assistant and do not interfere during the process.

   b. Address the issue based on the role the medical director is responsible to function in at that time.

   c. Most municipalities will have a conflict of interest policy which the medical director must comply with. If the agency lacks a formal policy, the medical director should reference the local or State policy.

Agency Oversight

Workforce Oversight and Supervision

One of the most important functions the medical director can perform is to have frequent quality interaction with the agency's emergency medical services (EMS) providers. EMS providers need to have ongoing interactions with the medical director, including education and mentoring, to ensure agency efficiency and provider effectiveness is optimized. These interactions allow the medical director to identify strengths that may take the organization in positive directions, and weaknesses that need to be remediated before they affect a patient. As previously mentioned, the medical director needs to make every reasonable effort to know all of their providers. In larger agencies, the medical director may also use the agency's chain of command to assist with the ongoing monitoring of all EMS providers.

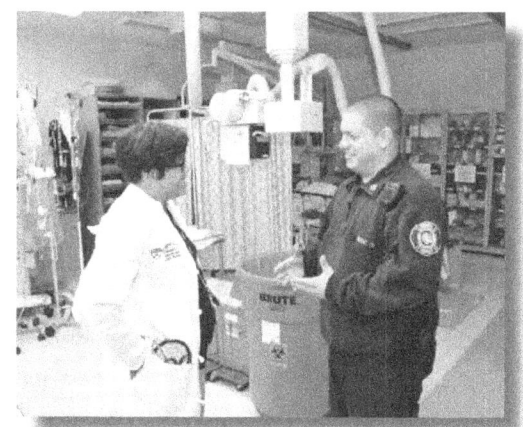

A medical director should provide essential:

* medical leadership;

* agency medical oversight;

* medical-related education and training, both initial, continuing, and refresher education;

* coordination of medical-related standard operating procedures (SOPs) and protocols;

* medical-related emergency preparedness and disaster care;

* implementation of medical-related best practices;

* medical-related quality improvement;

* provider health and safety measures; and

* research activities related to efficiency and efficacy of out-of-hospital patient care practices and patient outcomes.

According to the Institute of Medicine (IOM), some of the greatest challenges for the medical director related to EMS are

* Workforce shortages—Insufficient staffing of EMS resources due to inadequate compensation or difficult working conditions. Common EMS industry working conditions which can be classified as difficult are high-call volumes and long work hours.

* Lack of nationwide training requirements which cause wide variation in the quality of care—Stringent requirements related to training, certification, and licensing issues may impact EMS providers' ability to work in different regions, neighboring jurisdictions, or States.

* Occupational hazards that include infectious and contagious diseases, violence, and vehicle crashes—EMS activities are frequently performed in uncontrolled and unpredictable environments.

- Risk of terrorist incidents and lack of disaster preparedness—EMS providers are often first on the scene of all-hazard incidents including natural and manmade disasters. EMS providers are susceptible to dangers that other members of the health-care community may not be typically exposed to.

- The ability to care for pediatric patients—EMS providers respond to medical and traumatic incidents involving pediatric patients. Specialized training is required to adequately care for this subset of patients. Some EMS providers may have limited exposure to the pediatric population and some may not be as comfortable caring for pediatric patients as they are with the adult patients they routinely care for.

- Overcrowding of emergency departments—Emergency department overcrowding affects EMS agencies. Overcrowding can lead to long wait times for EMS resources to transfer care of their patients to the receiving hospital. Overcrowding may result in ambulances being diverted to other hospitals. Diversions from facilities with specialty services, such as a Level One Trauma Center, to a facility with lesser capabilities, can be detrimental to patient outcomes. Extended wait times can affect the operational capacity of the EMS system and cause resource availability shortages.

In addition to the challenges identified above, medical directors may also find that geriatric patients present specific challenges for an EMS agency. The geriatric patient population is one of the fastest growing subsets of patients and represents a disproportional incident volume when compared to any other age demographic set. Medical directors should ensure EMS providers receive initial and continuing education training in the emergency care of geriatrics.

Provisions of Patient Care

Protocols

Protocols help define the scope of out-of-hospital care for an EMS agency and prescribe recommended approaches for the provider to managing particular patient care situations.[16] In general, EMS providers must closely adhere to the protocols unless otherwise advised by online medical direction or clearly indicated by specific patient condition and reaction to usually employed therapies.[17] If online medical direction provides specific orders, the EMS provider must ensure to only perform those patient care treatments identified and approved within their level of certification or licensure.

In some systems, protocols may be developed and/or mandated by State or regional oversight entities. In these situations, protocol modifications by the local EMS agency's medical director may or may not be permitted. Systems may use locally developed protocols which can be created solely by the medical director or in collaboration with a crossfunctional committee within the agency and/or local medical community. In most cases, an agency's new medical director will choose to revise existing protocols rather than introducing a completely new protocol set. This approach may prove advantageous when limited advances in patient care standards are needed. All protocols deserve regular review and updates to reflect evidence-based changes in patient standard of care.

Standing Orders

Standing orders are more specific and are usually included within a protocol when a delay in treatment could be detrimental to the patient's medical condition.

Examples of standing orders for a paramedic may include

- defibrillation of a patient in ventricular fibrillation;
- advanced airway placement in an apneic patient; and
- medication administration for a cardiac arrest patient.

Protocols and standing orders should be evidence-based and be heavily guided by current peer-reviewed medical literature when available, evidence-based national standards, and State and regional patient care guidelines.[18] Often, these clinical directives must be carefully integrated into EMS industry operational practices themselves, subject to change based upon clinical advances.

Online Medical Direction

Online medical direction is the management of patient care by physicians through contact with the EMS providers by radio, phone, or other communication devices. EMS providers may seek online medical direction consultation to obtain orders, perform a procedure, or administer a drug that requires online approval. This communication allows for direct consultation on specific or unusual patient care situations and prepares the receiving facility for the incoming patient. This type of verbal communication may not always be given by the agency's medical director but by a physician at a designated medical facility.

Offline Medical Direction

Offline medical direction involves the development, dissemination, and enforcement of written instruction. Through offline medical direction, the EMS provider acts as an agent of the medical director.[19] Offline medical direction includes the administrative promulgation and enforcement of accepted standards for out-of-hospital care, including protocols and standing orders.

Offline medical direction can be accomplished through both prospective and retrospective methods. Prospective methods include, but are not limited to, training, provider testing and certification, protocol development, operational policy and procedures development, and legislative activities. Retrospective activities include, but are not limited to, medical audit and review of care, process improvement, direction of remedial education, and limitation of patient care functions.

Medical directors should actively participate in the agency's administration, education, quality improvement activities, and research endeavors that are critical to the success of the EMS agency. Committees with medical and provider representatives functioning under the medical director supervision can assist the medical director in performing various prospective and retrospective activities.

Medical Director in the Field

Medical directors should routinely participate in field responses, making first-hand contemporaneous patient care evaluations of the EMS system. This may take the form of ride-along experiences with EMS personnel to gain field experience, or may involve an individual response or response with an officer or other EMS entity within the agency. This activity will help evaluate the agency's effectiveness and the quality of service being rendered to ill and injured patients. The medical director's onscene observations and guidance on routine EMS responses will support a factual assessment of many aspects of service delivery, provide mentoring and coaching opportunities of EMS providers, and have the added benefit of demonstrating commitment to the EMS providers and agency leadership. Field exposure will also benefit the medical director in establishing initiatives that will advance their agency's performance, as well as provide evidence-based research opportunities in a clinical EMS setting. Although direct field experience with providers may be time-intensive, it is one of the most valuable experiences for both medical directors and providers.

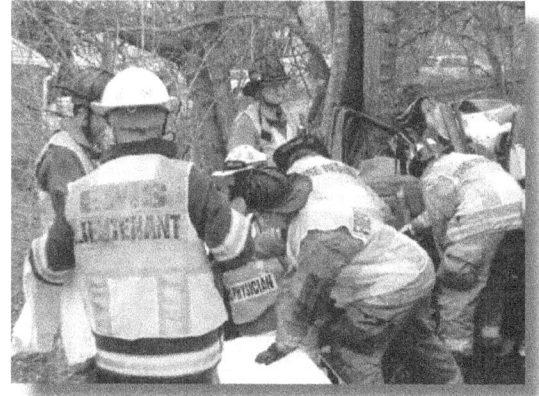

In some EMS agencies, the experienced and properly trained medical director not only observes, but also actively participates in out-of-hospital patient care on a regular basis. Often, these medical directors were themselves certified EMS providers prior to medical school. Indeed, the premise of the American Board of Medical Specialties' (ABMS') establishment of EMS as a medical subspecialty for physicians is that they will physically provide hands-on out-of-hospital patient care.

Medical directors need to have proper identification (e.g., agency identification cards, uniforms, etc.) and appropriate personal protective equipment (PPE) when participating in field operations.

Incident Command System

Whenever a medical director is participating with field operations, it is imperative that the Incident Command System (ICS) is understood and followed. This helps the medical director contribute to the management of the incident and not become a liability at the incident. The ICS is a standardized approach to manage emergency incidents and major events. The ICS is flexible and has a top-down organizational structure which begins when the first responder on the scene becomes the first Incident Commander (IC). The organizational structure can be expanded or contracted as necessary to accommodate the size of the incident.

When the medical director arrives on an emergency scene, they must immediately report to the Command Post for guidance, direction, and integration into the ICS, unless specifically directed to report to another area (e.g., Medical Branch or Staging) during their response to the incident scene. Properly trained medical directors can be of great value on the scene when they are fully integrated into the ICS.

Within the Incident Command structure, one of the possible medical functions is a Medical Branch. On-scene physicians often function as part of the Medical Branch or as a technical advisor to the IC. As resources arrive on the emergency scene, they are assigned to work in functional groups or geographic divisions and will report up the assigned chain of command.

The three functions in the Medical Branch are Triage, Treatment, and Transport. Triage is the rapid assessment and sorting of patients. There are several models that are widely accepted within the EMS industry. One model is the Centers for Disease Control and Prevention (CDC) Sort, Assess, Life-Saving Interventions, Treatment and/or Transport (SALT) triage method. SALT incorporates elements of other standardized methods of disaster triage. Another popular triage tool is the Simple Triage and Rapid Transport (START) model. The START triage model sorts patients into four color-coded categories:

Red (Immediate): Those with life threatening but treatable injuries who can be helped by *immediate* transportation.

Yellow (Delayed): Those with serious injuries but condition is stable enough for to have their transport *delayed*.

Green (Minimum): Those with minor injuries that can wait a longer time to be transported and need help less urgently.

Black (Deceased): Those who have injuries incompatible with life, or there is a lack of spontaneous respirations after the airway is opened.

Additional information regarding triage systems comparisons can be found at: www.dmphp.org/cgi/content/full/2/Supplement_1/S25

The Treatment Group is responsible for establishing the area to treat the patients that have been triaged. The treatment area will also be segregated by red, yellow, and green areas. EMS resources and equipment will be assigned to the various areas within the treatment area to initiate patient care and prepare patients for subsequent transport to medical facilities.

The Transportation Group coordinates the movement of patients from the treatment area to the receiving facilities.

EMS Scope of Practice

The "National EMS Scope of Practice Model (Scope of Practice)" divides the "National EMS Core Content" into four established provider levels, each with minimum skill and knowledge standards. As State EMS agencies begin to adopt the "National EMS Scope of Practice Model," it should be noted that the medical director may encounter providers using older terminology related to older scopes of practice levels.

- Emergency Medical Responder (EMR)--formerly known as First Responder;

- Emergency Medical Technician (EMT)--formerly known as EMT-Basic;

- Advanced Emergency Medical Technician (AEMT)--formerly known as EMT-Intermediate; and

- Paramedic--This term has remained the same.

The following descriptions are summaries from the "Scope of Practice" for the four established provider levels:

Emergency Medical Responder

The EMR possesses the basic knowledge and skills necessary to provide lifesaving interventions while awaiting arrival of additional EMS response resources. EMRs may assist higher-level certified EMS personnel at the scene and during patient transport. EMRs perform basic interventions such as basic patient assessment, oxygen administration, splinting, bandaging, and spinal immobilization with minimal equipment.

Emergency Medical Technician

The EMT possesses the basic knowledge and skills necessary to provided patient care and transportation. EMTs perform interventions with the basic equipment typically found on an ambulance. The EMT incorporates the skills of the EMR level but will have additional training related to patient assessment skills, gaining access to patients in various situations, ambulance operations, and will have clinical experience during their education program. In some States, the EMT may administer or assist with the administration of certain medications, use emergent airway adjuncts, and monitor existing intravenous fluid administration.

Advanced Emergency Medical Technician

The AEMT possesses all the knowledge and skills of the EMT. AEMTs can perform further skills such as intravenous or intraosseous fluid administration, certain advanced airway adjuncts, specific emergency care medications, and will have a greater depth and breadth of clinical procedure education as it relates to human anatomy and physiology.

Paramedic

The paramedic possesses the complex knowledge and skills necessary to provide advanced levels of patient care and transportation. The paramedic curriculum incorporates the EMR, EMT, and AEMT knowledge and skills, but also has additional hours of didactic and clinical requirements. The hourly requirements vary between States and programs, but paramedics usually have, at a minimum, approximately 1,000 additional educational hours above that of an EMT. The paramedic can be expected to perform advanced procedures such as endotracheal intubation, intravenous and intraosseous fluid administration, surgical airway techniques, medication administration related to several conditions, cardiac rhythm interpretation including 12-lead electrocardiograms (ECGs), defibrillation, and synchronized cardioversion, as well as other advanced procedures approved by the medical director.

Each educational level assumes mastery of previously stated competencies. Providers must demonstrate each competency within their scope of practice and for patients of all ages.[20] For a more detailed explanation related to the different EMS Scope of Practice for each can be found at EMS.gov at the following link: www.nhtsa.gov/people/injury/ems/EMSScope.pdf

The "Scope of Practice" determines what procedures a certified or licensed EMS provider is authorized to perform. This standard approach to identify provider levels supports the ability for States to uniformly recognize the certification or licensure levels, has the potential to resolve reciprocity issues between the States, and may assist in facilitating EMS provider mobility. However, at this time, the adoption of the "National EMS Scope of Practice Model" is not uniformly accepted by all States.

As previously mentioned, in States where the "Scope of Practice" is not accepted, there may be other governmental levels (State, regional, or locality) that establish and define the scope of practice for EMS providers. Adding to this variability is the issue that not all States use the National Registry of Emergency Medical Technicians (NREMT) certification exams, instead opting to develop their own testing for one or all of their certification or licensure levels. In these situations, a wide variety of provider titles and scope of practice definitions can exist. The medical director should become familiar with the current standards within their State. Additionally, it is crucial for the medical director to have knowledge of the EMS provider levels and associated skill sets within their agency.

Education Standards

National EMS Educational Standards

Often one of the medical director's responsibilities is the oversight of the EMS agency's educational programs. These educational programs may range from initial education of new providers, to the continuing education programs for incumbent providers within your agency. National Highway Traffic Safety Administration (NHTSA) has developed new "National EMS Educational Standards" according to each provider level. The medical director can view those standards and other related EMS issues (www.ems.gov).

The new "National EMS Educational Standards" will replace older EMS training curriculums and increase each provider-level standard for educational course development. The "National EMS Educational Standards" will be used as a basis for the development of new EMS textbooks by various publishers.

The basis for formulating the new "National EMS Educational Standards" originated from three published documents. The first document was titled the "Education Agenda," which had its roots in a document drafted in 1996 titled "The EMS Agenda for the Future." The "Education Agenda" called for a new and improved national EMS educational system that would work to increase efficiency and produce higher entry-level graduate competencies for EMS providers, as well as leading to national accreditation for EMS educational programs. The second document used to draft the new "National EMS Education Standards" comes from the "National EMS Core Content." This document lists all necessary course content to be provided in EMS education including patient conditions, chief complaints, operational issues, and provider psychomotor skills. The third document associated with this implementation of the new "National EMS Educational Standards" was the "National EMS Scope of Practice Model" published in 2005. This document identifies the four EMS personnel certification or licensure levels which were previously discussed in this chapter.

The "National EMS Educational Standards" define the competencies, clinical behaviors, and judgments that must be met by entry-level EMS personnel to meet practice guidelines defined in the "National EMS Scope of Practice Model."

The "National EMS Educational Standards" are made up of four components:

1. Competencies for each level of EMS provider (EMR, EMT, AEMT, and paramedic).

2. Knowledge required to achieve the competencies.

3. Clinical behaviors/judgments.

4. Educational infrastructure.

The "National EMS Educational Standards" provide a general framework to support individual programs for developing specific curricula to meet identified training and educational needs in particular regions. The format also allows for ongoing revision when research supports practice changes based on scientific evidence or when standards of care change. This approach is very different from previous approaches to curriculum development and revision which were infrequent and slowly implemented.

NHTSA has also published instructional guidelines for each provider certification level. These instructional guidelines include the basic information that programs must deliver in order for their students to meet the described competencies.

Medical directors are encouraged to engage with their State's EMS office to determine if these national standards will be adopted and identify associated implementation timelines.

Additionally, agencies providing certification courses will often need a physician course director. Each certification course will have its own set of defined physician oversight responsibilities and the medical director may want to also agree to serve in this capacity.

EMS Provider Continuing Education Program Development

The medical director needs to be involved in the development and approval of all agency-based continuing education initiatives to ensure the accuracy and validity of the courses' medical content. To address individual areas of concerns or agency trends, the medical director should incorporate findings from the agency's quality improvement initiatives into the continuing education program. There should be a seamless transition from the agency's quality improvement efforts to its education programs. Continuing education should be designed to meet three main objectives:

1. Provide exposure to current trends and evidence-based advances in patient care.

2. Review areas of patient assessment and management that are not frequently used.

3. Meet certification or licensure renewal requirements of the provider.

To ensure the developed continuing education program meets the providers' certification and/or licensing renewal criteria, agencies should have the course content verified by their State oversight agency or a nationally recognized entity. The Continuing Education Coordinating Board for Emergency Medical Services (CECBEMS) is a nationally recognized agency that will verify EMS continuing education course content. CECBEMS approved courses meet national standards and are generally accepted by NREMT.[21] Continuing education credits may also be obtained through other governmental agencies such as the Federal Emergency Management Agency (FEMA), if the course content is related to emergency response aspects. Medical directors should refer to their State EMS oversight agency for guidelines related to EMS continuing education programs and accepted credits.

In addition to their State certification or licensure, providers may also maintain certifications in various other training courses such as Advanced Cardiac Life Support (ACLS), Pediatric Advanced Life Support (PALS), International Trauma Life Support (ITLS), Prehospital Trauma Life Support (PHTLS), and Critical Care Emergency Medical Transport Program (CCEMTP). Medical directors may be requested to evaluate or support these courses as part of their provider credentialing process; therefore, the medical director will need to have a familiarization with training courses and their requirements.

Medical directors may need to work collaboratively with the agency's leadership on system design issues and assessments of provider certification levels to ensure requirements fit local needs and resources. These assessments will need to be periodically reviewed as the community's demographics may change or the EMS local environment becomes impacted by external forces. Examples of these situations may include single-level versus tiered system assessments or required transitions due to curriculum changes (e.g., discontinuation of NREMT—Intermediate level certification). Implementing system design changes will require modifications to provider initial and continuing education programs.

Provider Competency Verification

The medical director's role in oversight related to initial and continuing EMS education and competency is imperative to the success of the clinical application of out-of-hospital care by your agency. Of critical importance is the medical director's role in verifying all levels of providers' skill set competencies to ensure safe, efficient, and effective operational activities. Medical directors should have a direct role in the evaluation and refreshment of providers' skill sets. Competency assurance is verified by assessments of providers during the initial credentialing process and at periodic subsequent assessments. The assessments involve cognitive, psychomotor, and affective domains and are reflective of skills performed in the EMS profession. Low-frequency but high-criticality skills such as rapid sequence intubation, surgical airway procedures, and needle chest decompression are examples of procedures that will require frequent competency evaluations and educational support from the medical director to ensure providers remain ready to perform the skill in the out-of-hospital setting.

The task of competency verification can be accomplished in conjunction with your agency's training or operational staff. The medical director's oversight of competency-based evaluations may be identified in your agency's affiliation agreement, or may be a State or local EMS regulatory requirement.

Performance-Based Organizations

EMS is a multifaceted, integrated emergency response function that requires constant oversight. The medical director has the responsibility to assist their EMS agency with identifying improvements to patient care delivery processes, procedures, and equipment. By working cooperatively with agency leaders, supervisors, administrative specialists, and providers, the medical director can provide a team approach to manage the daily quality assessments of patient care-related activities to ensure that the EMS agency is operating effectively and providing the best prehospital care possible.

EMS agencies must be routinely evaluated for strengths, weaknesses, opportunities, and threats (SWOT) to have their policies and procedures revised to reflect best practices in the industry. The EMS agency's processes, equipment, and supplies should be routinely evaluated and considered for appropriate revisions and replacement to ensure EMS providers have the tools for performing their expected tasks.

Quality Improvement

A multitude of quality improvement (QI) activities have been performed by many EMS agencies through the history of EMS. In 1997, NHTSA produced a publication titled "A Leadership Guide to Quality Improvement in Emergency Medical Services (Leadership Guide)." The "Leadership Guide" was based largely on the seven Malcolm Baldridge Quality Categories:

1.   Leadership.

2.   Information and Analysis.

3.   Strategic Planning.

4.   Human Resource Development and Management.

5.   Process Management—Mapping.

6.   Agency Results.

7.   Stakeholder Satisfaction.

The "Leadership Guide" encouraged EMS leaders to integrate QI practices into daily EMS operations and organized performance measures into three developmental stages:

1.   Building potential for success by developing an awareness for QI.

2.   Expansion of QI knowledge, capabilities, and practices into agency workforce.

3.   Full integration of QI strategies into daily EMS operations.[22]

The medical director must have the authority to develop medical policies and procedures as well as the power to limit the actions of personnel who deviate from established standards. The medical director must also ensure that agency's protocols, procedures, and policies are consistent with their State's minimum requirements, including those for certification and/or licensure.

As one of the leaders in an EMS agency, the medical director should have authority over the agency's patient care quality management activities. EMS managers, supervisors, educators, providers, and external health-care community members must work together to accomplish quality management initiatives. The medical director needs to be involved in the development and monitoring of quality management related performance objectives in order to evaluate an agency's ability to meet its objectives. Quality management objectives can be developed from the following system components:

* communications;

* addressing complaints;

* documentation;

* reduction and prevention of illness and injury;

* patient confidentiality;

* performance objects;

* physician participation;

* public health outcome parameters; and

* participation in studies and research.[23,24]

Types of Quality Improvement

QI may be prospective, concurrent, or retrospective in nature. EMS providers and supervisors should be held accountable for the procedures that the medical director and agency leadership have put in place. EMS agencies should conduct their QI program using components of all of the types of QI mechanisms listed below. EMS providers and other end users need to be involved in the process. QI activities should not be designed to be punitive in nature for individual providers but instead be focused on organizational improvements and conducted to educate providers and ultimately enhance patient care delivery.

Prospective Improvement

Prospective QI may be in the form of primary education of EMS personnel, continuing education, periodic skill evaluation, and training programs. This type of improvement is seen as a front-end approach to improvement.

Concurrent Improvement

Concurrent QI is achieved through direct observation of performance of EMS providers at the time of service provision. Most EMS agencies have a chain of command that includes EMS supervisors or officers that conduct direct oversight and leadership of providers. Direct supervision or oversight on the scene of a cardiac arrest or an automobile collision by a medical director or EMS officer is an example of concurrent QI.

Retrospective Improvement

Retrospective QI may be in the form of documentation, case reviews, or audits. Patient care records can be checked for completeness and accuracy in order to determine the level of compliance with established agency policies and protocols. Retrospective QI involves activities that look back to see if quality service was provided. Review of patient care records, response surveys mailed to patients and families, interface with other EMS responder agencies, surveys of receiving hospitals, response time studies, and high-risk call reviews are reflective of retrospective QI.[25,26]

Figure 1 is an example of all three types of current QI models found in an effective EMS QI program.

Figure 1: Example of Quality Improvement[27]

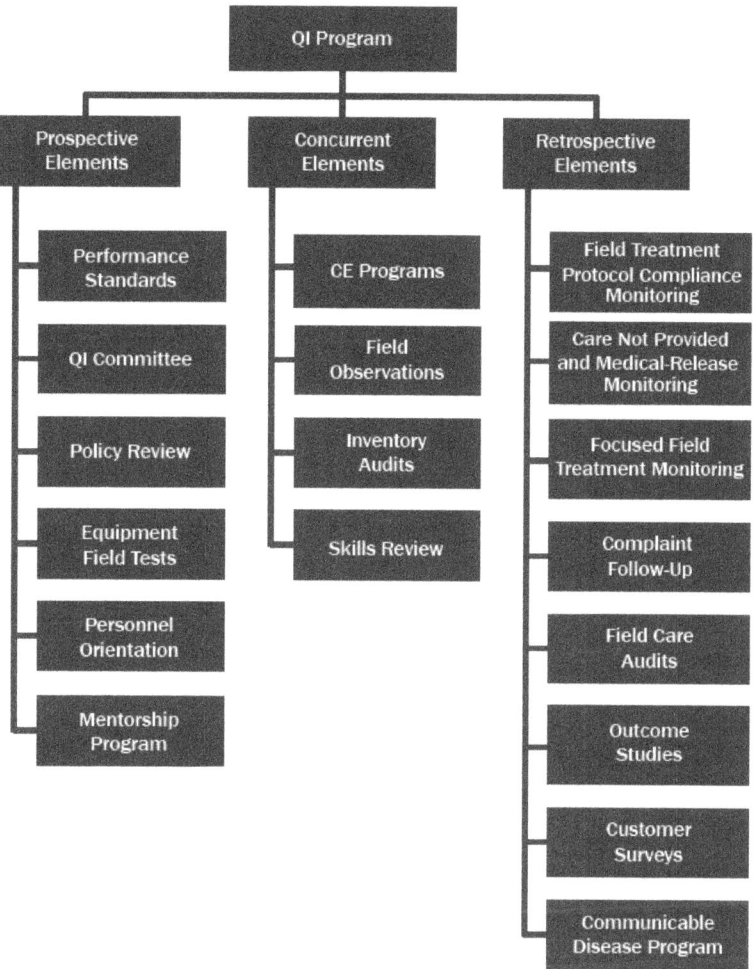

Six Sigma in EMS

Six Sigma is a process improvement methodology approach that focuses on the ability to reduce variation. The concept and training program was originally developed by Bill Smith at Motorola in 1986 and represented more than 60 years of QI practices.[28] This philosophical approach has been well used in the retail and manufacturing sector, but EMS agencies are adapting the process to their environment. Examples of agencies using this process are Lee County, FL and Memphis, TN. There are several books on the market related to this method and variations of this method, like Lean Six Sigma, that meets the service industries needs for quality management. It should be noted that there are other quality improvement approaches and tools. Like the Six Sigma method, most are nonproprietary.

The basis of Six Sigma is the usage of data and statistical analysis to identify and modify processes within an organization or project team. Six Sigma incorporates a top-down approach where quality is owned by everyone and directed by those in top management. Process improvement where Six Sigma can be of assistance may include

- hiring processes;

- QI processes;

- response times;

- offload times at hospitals;

- revenue recovery; and

- customer satisfaction.

Six Sigma can assist with prioritizing, selecting, supporting, and managing QI initiatives in all aspects of an organization.[29]

HIPAA and Quality Improvement

The Health Insurance Portability and Accountability Act of 1996 (HIPAA) enacted Federal protections for personal health information. The increased privacy protection awareness and regulations can result in some covered entities not recognizing EMS as a vital link in the patient's progression through the health-care system. EMS records need to be linked with hospital records in order to support patient outcome data that a medical director will need to perform comprehensive QI activities.

QI measures are subject to HIPAA's minimum necessary standard. This means that only the minimum amount of information necessary to conduct a quality review or consultation on the incident should be disclosed. Copies of patient care documentation used in case review activities must have all nonessential information redacted, such as the patient's name and address.

To avoid difficulties in performing patient followup and outcome activities with receiving facilities, it is recommended that the medical director assist in facilitating the need for the agency's QI program manager to obtain contact points at each receiving facility for this purpose. Multidimensional case reviews with providers, emergency department staff, and agency leaders will assist in discovering potential QI opportunities.

Performance Measures

Agency evaluation using performance measures can be imperative in the overall quality and effectiveness assessment of an EMS agency, particularly if the performance measure has been validated by peer-reviewed and evidence-based literature. A performance measure is a quantifiable criterion that relates to program quality. Internally, these indicators can be used as a quality evaluation and planning tool to determine and track agency activities.[30] Externally, the indicators can be used as comparative and objective measures across different agencies. An ideal measure is one that is not only quantifiable, but one that has been shown to make differences in patient outcomes. It should be noted that a clinically relevant "best practices" approach should be used related to performance measures until true evidence is accumulated. Examples of performance measures used in QI activities are

- turn out times for response vehicles;

- distance or locations of EMS units; and

- time to treatment for time-sensitive clinical conditions (e.g., time of patient contact to ECG acquisition time in ST segment elevation myocardial infarction (STEMI) patients).

  International Association of Fire Fighters (IAFF)/International Association of Fire Chiefs (IAFC) EMS System Performance Measurement

  Together, the IAFF and the IAFC constructed, field-tested, validated, and published an EMS System Performance Measurement instrument in 2002. This instrument consists of 15 EMS quality indicators, definitions, and related performance measures. The publication provides background information relating each indicator to the overall quality assessment of an EMS agency. The document also explains existing standards (or lack thereof), potential agency goals, and identifies needed data collection related to each measure.[31] A sample of the performance measures can be referenced in Appendix H.

Meyers et al., *Prehosp Emerg Care: Evidence-Based Performance Measures for Emergency Medical Services Systems*

In 2007, the U.S. Metropolitan Municipalities' EMS Medical Directors' Consortium developed and published evidence-based performance measures for EMS systems. These performance measures include a broad base of clinical situations and discuss EMS interventions. A sample of these outcome-centric benchmarks can be referenced in Appendix H.

Several other organizations have also participated in efforts to establish consensus standards for quality measurement in EMS. These organizations include National Fire Protection Association (NFPA) (NFPA 450, *Guide for Emergency Medical Services and Systems*), NHTSA ("EMS Performance Measures—Recommended Attributes and Indicators for System and Service Performance"), Commission on Accreditation of Ambulance Services (CAAS), American Society for Testing and Materials (ASTM) F-30, American Heart Association (AHA), as well as local and State health authorities.[32] Medical directors are encouraged to use all of these resources to aid in their understanding of the concepts and assist with the implementation of QI and performance measure activities.

Benchmarking

Benchmarking is the practice of setting targets for a particular function by evaluating other related performers, either within or outside an organization. In a broader sense, benchmarking involves looking for and using new ideas and best practices for the improvement of processes, products, and services.

Unfortunately, there are tremendous gaps in data collection, QI, and benchmarking practices in the EMS industry. There are real and perceived barriers involved in this situation which have contributed to poor industry-level outcome tracking and wide variances in data availability to perform benchmarking activities. These barriers can include an agency's existing information management systems, data collection practices, and difficulties in gathering and assimilating clinical information as the patient travels through the healthcare continuum. These factors have contributed to EMS strategies, ranging from agency model development to patient treatment activities, having questionable benefit in overall patient outcomes. Many EMS practices have evolved from tradition or nonconventional application of in-hospital care modalities.

A needed component in addressing this industry information gap is the standardization of data elements so that EMS databases at all levels (local, regional, State, and Federal) can be linked. NHTSA, in coordination with the Health Resources and Services Administration, has developed the National EMS Information System (NEMSIS) which includes a national EMS database and data definitions that can be used for the evaluation of patient and agency outcomes, be a source for benchmarking performance, and facilitate the development of industry research and training curriculums.[33] The majority of States have agreed to participate with the project but their implementation timelines vary. In order to understand how the NEMSIS project is impacting a medical director's agency, the medical director should contact their State EMS oversight agency for additional information. The following website is a useful source for information on NEMSIS: www.nemsis.org

As the EMS industry continues to evolve, performance documentation will be critical to demonstrate system effectiveness. In the interim, medical directors should establish collaborative relationships with other medical directors in their region and State. Medical directors may also find particular value with establishing these relationships with other similar size and demographically equivalent agencies in order to perform benchmarking activities.

When performing benchmarking, a medical director needs to decide what information and data will be used during the process. The process needs to begin with evaluating your agency's performance measures. Performance measures identify your agency's accomplishments and benchmarking that information to other agencies' outcomes can be a beneficial exercise in QI efforts.

Benchmarking efforts often use data elements such as work schedules, response times, and number of specific patient care encounters (e.g., cardiac arrests). The medical director should not focus only on time-centered measures, such as how fast the agency arrives and the length of transport times as examples. The medical director should work with the agency's leadership to determine all aspects of EMS service delivery to identify where benchmarking may help to improve their agency's performance. These efforts will assist the medical director in ensuring the EMS agency is providing a quality and highly-valued service which is meeting system expectations and demands.

Best Practices

Closely related to benchmarking activities is the understanding of the EMS industry's best practices. Researching best practices can aid a medical director in their decisionmaking in the multidimensional environment they operate in. The best practice techniques, processes, methods, and policies can assist the medical director in implementing new initiatives with fewer complications, or in refining existing practices.

There are a multitude of sources where a medical director can research EMS industry best practices. Professional organizations and associations such as the American College of Emergency Physicians (ACEP), National Association of State EMS Officials (NASEMSO), National Association of EMS Physicians (NAEMSP), NFPA, IAFC, IAFF, NAEMT, International Association of EMS Chiefs (IAEMSC), National EMS Manager's Association (NEMSMA), as well as State EMS offices, and other local EMS agencies are all sources for information. Journals and industry periodicals will publish information vital to a medical director's decisionmaking considerations and be a source of consolidated research on a given topic. Best practices are available for equipment-related issues, training and education programs, testing environments, patient care-related activities, and QI initiatives.

The National Fire Academy (NFA) in Emmitsburg, MD, offers several operational and managerial courses in which are open to all service delivery models of EMS and are free of charge. One emerging course that applies to the improvement of service delivery in EMS is the *Emergency Medical Services: Quality Management* (EMS:QM). Information pertaining to NFA EMS courses can be found at:

www.usfa.dhs.gov/nfa

www.usfa.dhs.gov/media/press/2011releases/012711.shtm

Ambulance Service Accreditation

A mechanism to recognize an agency's efforts and accomplishments is to consider pursuing accreditation for their EMS agency. Standards for accreditation are designed to increase operational efficiency and clinical quality, and decrease risk and liability to your organization.[34] The CAAS, the Center for Public Safety Excellence (CPSE), and the Commission on Accreditation of Medical Transport Systems (CAMTS) are industry organizations that recognize emergency service best practices through their accreditation processes. There are numerous benefits for an agency, regardless of the agency type (e.g., fire-based, private) to achieve accreditation, including positive public perceptions, an external validation for local officials and the medical community that the agency underwent careful review, and recognition of the efforts of all personnel affiliated with the agency. Efforts to obtain and maintain accreditation status is another area where the medical director must cooperatively work with agency leadership to achieve this goal.

EMS Research

EMS is in its relative infancy as an industry and as a method of delivering health-care services. Research activities in EMS are progressing, but have historically been recognized as one of the weaknesses in refining patient care and systems design in EMS. Several EMS research initiatives related to medications, equipment, and treatment modalities are underway and have the potential to influence the EMS patient care delivery arena. A medical director should use the results of evidenced-based EMS research to evaluate and adjust clinical practices, equipment usage, and the delivery of EMS services. The medical director should use regular journal reviews and continuing education opportunities to stay abreast of developments in research and patient care that could influence prehospital care. The medical director should also consider the involvement of their agency in appropriate research studies and pilot programs to further advance EMS care.[35] The NFA also has a *Hot Topics Research in EMS* course that medical directors may be interested in. Additional information can be found at: www.usfa.dhs.gov/nfa

Health and Safety of Medical Directors and Providers

The medical director should be an advocate for health and safety issues and for safer workplace practices. The Occupational Safety and Health Administration (OSHA), a regulatory agency in of the Department of Labor (DOL), works to ensure safe working conditions for personnel by establishing and enforcing standards, as well as providing workforce education and training. OSHA provides workforce oversight either directly through the Federal organization or through an approved State program. Medical directors should become familiar with applicable OSHA standards for EMS and have knowledge of their State's program if applicable, as well as understand the agency's investigative and enforcement procedures. The medical director needs to understand that their patient care oversight responsibilities are distinctively different than the agency's occupational physician's role and responsibility for the agency is. Typically, these two services are not provided by the same physician.

NFPA also publishes industry standards related to various EMS-related situations. One such standard that addresses personnel's minimum requirements for performing roles within an all-hazard Incident Management System (IMS) is NFPA 1026, *Standard for Incident Management Personnel Professional Qualifications*. Medical directors may also want to become familiar with other applicable NFPA standards.

The medical director also needs an appreciation for the physical and mental toll that extended operations can have on emergency workers. NFPA 1584, *Standard on the Rehabilitation Process for Members During Emergency Operations and Training Exercises* identifies the minimum criteria for establishing a rehabilitation process for personnel operating at incident scene operations and training exercises, and is a document that the medical director should reference.

The use of personal safety equipment is vital to protection and safety against exposure to infection. Proper application of PPE and body substance isolation (BSI) is a cornerstone for medical director and EMS providers' safety. Appropriate use of BSI for the given situation should be a mandate for EMS providers.

The compromised use of PPE during emergency incidents or training evolutions can lead to injury or even death of the EMS provider. Personnel without appropriate levels of PPE must not be permitted to operate during emergencies or training events. Despite being intensely focused on the medical care of patients, EMS providers must wear appropriate PPE to protect against cutting forces, falling objects, exposures, and other scene hazards. An example of certain PPE specified by regulations and statues is the requirement of EMS providers to wear a high-visibility vest during roadway incident operations to aid in their visibility to other rescuers and civilians. This high-visibility clothing must meet the requirements of American National Standards Institute (ANSI)/International Safety Equipment Association (ISEA) 107; 2004 edition Class 2 or 3.[36] Additionally, NFPA 1500, *Standard on Fire Department Occupational Safety and Health Program* and NFPA 1999, *Standard on Protective Clothing for Emergency Medical Operations* should be used as a guideline for protection of prehospital providers.

Areas of safety concern should include, but not be limited to:

- head and face protection;

- ear and hearing protection;

- hand protection;

- foot protection; and

- body protection.

A health and safety area that is receiving considerable attention is the development and design of ambulances and equipment. These issues will be discussed later in the handbook, but medical directors must recognize these issues not only impact provider safety but impact the safety of the public at large. The development of dispatch and patient care protocols that also address response vehicle operations is another area for the medical director's attention and involvement.

Patient Safety

Patients also need to be shielded from the same incident elements that providers are also being exposed to. Examples of items that will help to create a safe environment for patients are

- blankets for warmth and debris protection;

- helmet;

- hearing protection;

- goggles;

- dust mask, unless patient is having difficulty breathing and/or is on oxygen; and

- shielding devices such as backboards placed to form a barrier between the patient and sharp objects or equipment.[37]

The health and safety of providers needs to be a paramount concern and a responsibility shared by every member and supervisory level in an agency. In addition to the resources discussed in the section, there are several other professional nongovernment organizations and government agencies identified in the handbook that have safety-related information and resources (e.g., IAFC, IAFF, NHTSA, U.S. Fire Administration (USFA), Department of Health and Human Services (HHS), CDC, OSHA, National Institute for Occupational Safety and Health (NIOSH), National Volunteer Fire Council (NVFC)).

Agency Dynamics

A medical director has responsibility for the oversight of many multifaceted and dynamic aspects of an emergency medical services (EMS) agency. Medical directors must understand the wide depth and breadth of involvement as it relates to interacting and interfacing with your EMS agency, its leadership, and its many providers. Understanding the medical director's role is crucial to success, both at the individual and agency levels.

Ambulance Service Certificate of Need

A medical director may become involved in the implementation of a new EMS agency or a planned expansion of an existing EMS agency. The medical director, along with the EMS agency leaders, must comply with any applicable State and local regulations related to the establishment and expansion of an EMS agency.

In some States, EMS agencies may be required to obtain a Certificate of Need for their agency startup or planned expansion. If applicable, the Certificate of Need process can be found in State and/or local statues. This process is designed to identify the geographic area in which the agency may operate, identify the type of service to be provided, and provide authorization for the service to begin operations. The Certificate of Need process is not uniformly required across all regions and/or States. The medical director must check with the appropriate local, regional, and State entities to determine what governmental regulations may be related to EMS agency licensing and operations.

As EMS authorizing agencies vary from State to State, it is challenging to address each States' regulating authority to the reader in general terms. Some States have very involved EMS regulatory offices with robust authority, while others have little authority and responsibility and is quite localized. As will be pointed out several times within this handbook, the medical director must understand how systems operate within their State and understand the regulating authority's role.

Public Relations

Media Inquiries

The medical director is viewed by both the media and the public as a trusted official who needs to be concerned with the quality of their EMS agency's performance and must be highly responsive to inquiries. Establishing positive media relations is important for an EMS agency and the medical director. There are numerous ethical and legal considerations which must be evaluated when preparing and releasing media responses. These considerations include the Health Insurance Portability and Accountability Act of 1996 (HIPAA) related issues, protecting investigative information from premature release, and the Freedom of Information Act (FoIA) related issues. While some EMS agencies may have a public relations office or officer that can assist the medical director, it is critical that the medical director work in concert with the agency's leadership to coordinate responses to all media requests for information. Medical directors may not have previous experience with media relations and this may be an area that medical directors request specific agency-level training.

EMS Advocacy

Medical directors should take an active role in promoting their EMS agency and being an advocate for the overall EMS industry. The medical director position is dynamic and will include interactions with many external system stakeholders. The medical director can be an effective liaison to these external stakeholders and leverage a great deal of credibility in communicating EMS agency accomplishments and needs. The medical director should coordinate these advocacy activities with the agency's leadership to achieve a shared, consistent message and to increase the effectiveness of efforts.

Advocacy activities may involve public speaking appearances to city or county governmental or elected officials in an attempt to articulate local EMS agency needs and service delivery issues, provide budget justifications, and describe the impact of State and local EMS rules and regulations. The advocacy role will certainly require the medical director to interact with other health-care professionals, public health officials, and members of other emergency service agencies to promote and coordinate the involvement of the EMS agency as an active partner in the emergency response and medical community.

Credentialing in EMS

Another aspect of the medical director's oversight is verification of your EMS providers' credentials. The medical director may seek assistance with this function within the administrative staff of their agency. Specific items related to EMS credentialing vary from region to region and State to State. As previously discussed in the handbook, some States may license providers while other States will certify them. The medical director should check with the State EMS office for additional guidance. EMS personnel education and training history, licensure or certification history, active or nonactive status, and general contact information may need to be available for credential review by State or regional EMS offices.

EMS Education Program Dynamics

Accreditation of Education Programs

The "EMS Agenda for the Future" recommended a single national accreditation agency for all EMS certification levels be established. Yet, not all levels of EMS education programs have a national requirement to be an accredited program. Currently, there are no national level accreditation requirements for educational programs below the level of paramedic. In November 2007, the National Registry of Emergency Medical Technicians (NREMT) Board of Directors implemented a new requirement that in order to be eligible to attempt the NREMT testing and credentialing process, all paramedic applicants must have graduated from an accredited program.

This requirement has a targeted effective date of January 1, 2013. Paramedics who are certified prior to January 1, 2013, will be "grandfathered" and are not impacted by this new requirement. Once again, the medical director needs to check with their State's EMS oversight agency to receive guidance on any State-level requirements for educational programs since not all States use NREMT testing for all or any level of EMS provider.

If an agency has an initial training program for the paramedic certification level, or is seeking to establish this type of program, the medical director should seek educational program accreditation to ensure national educational standards are met. The Commission on Accreditation of Allied Health Education Programs (CAAHEP), through its Committee on Accreditation of Educational Programs for the Emergency Medical Services Professions (CoAEMSP), is the only national agency that offers EMS paramedic education program accreditation.

Though the CoAEMSP standards and guidelines may be adopted for the education infrastructure section of a paramedic educational program, this does not mean the program is CoAEMSP accredited. At present, some paramedic programs may only have a State approval process, but not a CoAEMSP accreditation requirement.

For most EMS educational programs, the medical director should commit a significant amount of time to the program, for which appropriate compensation is often necessary. To meet CoAEMSP standards, the medical director must

- be a physician currently licensed to practice medicine within the United States and currently authorized to practice within the geographic area served by the program, with experience and current knowledge of emergency care of acutely ill and injured patients;

- have adequate training or experience in the delivery of out-of-hospital emergency care, including the proper care and transport of patients, medical direction, and quality improvement (QI) in out-of-hospital care;

- be an active member of the local medical community and participate in professional activities related to out-of-hospital care; and

- be knowledgeable about the education of the Emergency Medical Services Professions, including professional, legislative, and regulatory issues regarding the education of the Emergency Medical Services Professions.

In addition, the medical director must be responsible for all medical aspects of the program, including, but not limited to:

- review and approval of the educational content of the program curriculum to certify its ongoing appropriateness and medical accuracy;

- review and approval of the quality of medical instruction, supervision, and evaluation of the students in all areas of the program;

- review and approval of the progress of each student throughout the program and assist in the development of appropriate corrective measures when a student does not show adequate progress;

- assurance of the competence of each graduate of the program in the cognitive, psychomotor, and affective domains;

- responsibility for cooperative involvement with the program director; and

- adequate controls to assure the quality of the delegated responsibilities.[38]

CoAEMSP standards and guidelines regarding the role of the medical director can be obtained from their website: www.coaemsp.org/Documents/Standards.pdf

Certification of Providers

Following the successful completion of an approved EMS educational program, the prospective EMS provider is eligible to attempt certification and/or licensing testing. The battery of testing is both didactic and practical in nature. This process provides verification that an individual possesses the necessary knowledge and skills to perform at the provider's certification level.[39]

The NREMT is the national testing body for the provider levels identified in the "National EMS Scope of Practice Model." NREMT facilitates certification by conducting standardized registration and testing (written and practical exams). NREMT is recognized by most, but not all States. Currently, 46 States use the NREMT for testing one or more EMS certification levels. States that do not use the NREMT must use their own developed testing requirements, which may not be recognized by other States. This variability leads to inconsistency, lack of reciprocity, and is incongruent with recommendations contained in the "Education Agenda." During their 2010 annual meeting, the National Association of State EMS Officials (NASEMSO) adopted a resolution supporting NREMT as the national EMS certification agency, and CoAEMSP as the National EMS education program accreditation agency.

Each State's EMS oversight agency has the right to certify and/or license EMS providers, including if they elect to use NREMT certification. The medical director should become familiar with related certification practices and requirements within their State.

Recertification of EMS Providers

Continuing education is a requirement for recertification and/or licensure renewal for all levels of EMS providers. Each provider level is required to complete a specified number of continuing education hours, depending on State and/or NREMT requirements. The length of time for recertification and/or licensure renewal varies among the States and typically ranges between 2 to 3 years. NREMT has a 2-year recertification period.

Recertification requires continuing education and competency verification. Medical directors must again become familiar with related certification and recertification requirements within their State. Listed below are examples of NREMT recertification requirements which most States use for initial certification and recertification.

NREMT Biennial Recertification Requirements

Emergency Medical Responder (EMR) Recertification Requirements

- The EMR can recertify through two different options:

    - traditional refresher course—an approved Department of Transportation (DOT) National Standard Emergency Responder Refresher or Continuing Education Coordinating Board for Emergency Medical Services (CECBEMS) approved refresher course; or

    - continuing education topical hours—a refresher may be completed by attending continuing education classes which cover the required topics and hours.

- Submission of approved cardiopulmonary resuscitation (CPR) certification.

- Obtain verification of skill competence by medical director or training program director.

- Pay a recertification application fee.

Emergency Medical Technician (EMT) Recertification Requirements

- Complete a total of 72 hours of education which consists of:

    - an approved 24-hour DOT National Standard EMT Refresher Course or continuing education hours, specifically meeting the refresher curriculum objectives; and

    - complete 48 hours of additional continuing EMS-related education.

- Submission of approved CPR certification.

- Obtain verification of skill competence by medical director or training program director.

- Pay a recertification application fee.

Advanced EMT Recertification Requirements

- Complete a total of 72 hours of education which consists of:

    - an approved 36-hour refresher course or continuing education hours specifically meeting the refresher curriculum objectives; and

    - complete 36 hours of additional continuing EMS-related education.

- Submission of approved CPR certification.

- Obtain verification of skill competence by medical director or training program director.

- Pay a recertification application fee.

Paramedic Recertification Requirements

- Complete a total of 72 hours of education which consists of:

    - an approved 48-hour DOT National Standard Paramedic Refresher or continuing education hours, specifically meeting the refresher curriculum objectives; and

    - complete 24 hours of additional continuing EMS-related education.

- Submission of approved Advanced Cardiac Life Support (ACLS) and CPR certification.

- Obtain verification of skill competence by medical director or training program director.

- Pay a recertification application fee.

Exam Option—Certified EMS providers may make one attempt to demonstrate continued cognitive competency by taking an examination in lieu of documenting continuing education. The exam attempt must be made 6 months prior to their certification expiration date.

Agency Compliance Considerations

Collective Bargaining Agreements

Collective bargaining is a process of negotiations between employers and labor unions to achieve workplace agreements. Items that are typically discussed and collectively bargained include wage compensation, work hours, health and safety, occupational environment, benefits, and union and management rights. In addition, procedures to resolve disputes and grievances may also be bargained. The resulting agreement will be a written collective agreement, contract, or memorandum of understanding (MOU) between the employee union, which acts as the bargaining agent, and the employer. In some States, collective bargaining may involve binding arbitration. In these areas, when negotiation efforts fail, the process may reach impasse. At this point, employees and employers must present their items of interests (e.g., safety issues) to a neutral arbitrator or arbitration panel for a decision. Based on local or State laws, the arbitrator's decision may be binding on both parties. The resulting decision then becomes part of the collective agreement, contract, or MOU that is effectively a legal document.

The medical director will need to establish a productive working dialogue and relationship with all work representative groups within an agency. There is also a need to have a basic understanding of any collective bargaining agreements that may be in place.

In addition to understanding employer/employee agreements, the medical director also needs a clear understanding of his/her role in provider oversight as it relates to patient care delivery activities. There may be instances such as QI initiatives that could result in the remediation or training enhancement of an EMS provider. It is important for the medical director, the employee, and the union to understand that while they are responsible to patients for providing the highest quality of available care, they are also committed to fostering a productive work environment in which to deliver that care. Issues related to the oversight role of the medical director and the relation to any progressive discipline procedures are discussed in the Becoming a Medical Director chapter of this handbook.

Federal, State, and local legislation provisions need to be reviewed as they relate to mandated or formal QI programs. The medical director should seek out union assistance and interact professionally in establishing the understanding of the medical director's medical oversight mission. Any service delivery-related medical practices and/or policies that a medical director desires to institute should be clearly articulated verbally and in writing, and be open for discussion prior to final implementation.

Right to Work States

In 22 States, there is a Right to Work law. Right to Work laws permit individuals to decide if they prefer to join or financially contribute to a union. In these States, employees cannot be required to join or pay dues to a labor union. In these States, if an individual elects to have joined a union but then later decides to resign from their union, they can still be covered by the collective bargaining agreement that was in place during their membership time period. The medical director needs to understand the labor environment their agency operates in to avoid any potential conflicts and establish the appropriate professional relationships.

Industry Regulations and Standards

As previously discussed in the EMS Agency and Its Stakeholder chapter of this handbook, the medical director must be aware of entities that produce industry regulations, standards, and guidelines affecting EMS providers and agencies. Two of the most commonly referenced agencies are Occupational Safety and Health Administration (OSHA) and National Fire Protection Association (NFPA). These organizations and the documents they produce can assist the medical director in fostering a healthy and safe working environment for their providers. The medical director must be aware that OSHA regulations are enforceable by law but the NFPA produces industry standards and guidelines that should be considered for adoption by the EMS agency. Appendix G contains selected examples that apply to common conditions applicable to emergency response agencies including EMS.

Fiscal Management Issues

Budgeting

Regardless of if your EMS agency is public, private, for-profit, or nonprofit, it will have a budgetary process that provides the agency's fiscal management plan. How the EMS agency's leadership manages its budget will dictate the agency's long-term viability. The agency's budget should be a driving force for what is monitored and to aid decisionmaking on a daily basis. The budget process can be helpful with:

*   monitoring of day-to-day operations;

*   resource for planning activities;

*   aid in the identification of organizational sentinel events; and

*   facilitates evaluation and selection of potential solutions based on data.[40]

The medical director needs to cooperatively work with the EMS agency's leadership in the budgetary planning process by projecting program needs and costs to facilitate the development of a comprehensive financial plan.

Federal and State Funding Sources

Federal level funding is typically distributed to States and may be further passed on to localities. Many States allocate funding for State oversight agencies and local EMS agencies through a variety of general fund allocations, administration of grant programs, or incentive programs that return a portion of collected taxes or fees back to the locality. Some of the funding sources that are available for EMS activities at the Federal and State levels include

*   vehicle-related registration fees;

*   traffic enforcement-related fees;

- health and/or homeowner's insurance surcharges;

- grant programs; and

- general fund revenue allocations.

Local Funding Sources

Local funding sources can also be derived from a variety of sources. Listed below are some general categories that localities will often have as funding sources:

- Taxes—General property, local income, sales, and district taxes. This is the most common source of municipality-controlled funding for EMS agencies.

- Fees—These include fees for construction-related permits, special events permits, hazardous use permits, facility inspections, and building or life safety code violations.

- Fines and citations—Agencies may charge fees for actions that are inconsistent with the law, such as traffic enforcement fines.

- Development impact fees—New developments may be required to pay for the impact the development will have on the locality's capital outlays such as new fire station construction and associated equipment purchases.

- Revenue recovery—Billing third-party insurance companies to recover reimbursement allowed for EMS transport services. Reimbursement rates will be based on the level of service provided and mileage traveled.

- Subscriptions—An annual fee paid to an EMS agency to offset any insurance copayments so there are no out-of-pocket costs incurred by the patient.

- Benefit assessment charges—Administered similar to property taxes, these charges are based on factors such as being located in close proximity to fire stations, having reduced insurance rates, or the availability of special services.

- Strategic alliances—Agencies may form alliances and partnerships with other agencies to provide services under an annual contract with associated fees.

- Grants—Governmental and private entity grants exist.

- Sales of assets and services—Agencies may sell used equipment or services.

Agency-Level Funding Sources

Career and volunteer fire and EMS agencies may raise a significant amount of funds from the private sector. Agencies are increasingly turning to private donations, often by setting up nonprofit foundations. Private sector funding sources include the following:

- private foundations;

- corporate donations; and

- public and private partnerships.

Revenue Recovery Sources

Many EMS agencies have instituted revenue recovery programs in which insurance companies, including Medicare and Medicaid, are billed for EMS transport services. Costs of emergency care are already included in actuarial calculations of insurance premiums and are a viable revenue source for EMS agencies.

Medicare and Medicaid, as a means for generating revenue for the agency, can only be billed by transporting EMS agencies for the level of care administered during the patient transport and mileage traveled with the patient onboard. Agencies may perform their own billing services or contract with a billing services company. If a billing contractor is used, the billing company will charge a fee which is typically a percentage of the collected revenue. Fee percentages as well as the billing company's collection practices are negotiated contractual items with the EMS agency. Medical directors should be very familiar with the agency's policies and procedures for billing insurance companies including their role, if any, in any signoff or review procedures.

Funding for Medical Directors

Funding for medical oversight activities, when the oversight is not provided on a volunteer basis, can come from a variety of sources which may include the following:

*   Hospital or physician practice groups may provide financial and administrative support for the EMS medical director.

*   Agency dedicated funding for medical director compensation.

Apparatus and Equipment

Ambulance Design

To ensure safety for both EMS providers and patients in ambulances, there are industry standards that address ambulance design and construction. Currently, the most popular ambulance specifications are the Federal KKK-A-1822 standard and the National Truck Equipment Association Ambulance Manufacturers Division standard (2007 version). Ambulance design is currently undergoing a period of increased interest and scrutiny with the goal being to increase the safety of patients and providers. Recently, the NFPA has formed a multidisciplinary committee to develop a new ambulance design standard for the EMS industry. This new standard will replace the existing KKK-A-1822 specifications and will address the design, construction, and testing requirements for ambulances. The new standard will be NFPA 1917, *Standard for Automotive Ambulances* and is expected to be published in 2013.

EMS Equipment and Technology

EMS equipment is specially designed to be compact, portable, durable, and lightweight, and technology is ever-evolving and becoming more sophisticated. The type and minimum amount of equipment required for both basic life support (BLS) and advanced life support (ALS) transport vehicles is regulated by the State in which the ambulance operates.

Computers, cell phones, Bluetooth, and other technology have also revolutionized EMS care. Not only has technology helped save patients' lives, it is also beginning to improve data capturing and reporting processes. Some EMS agencies have implemented, or plan to implement, electronic patient care reporting systems. When an EMS agency is capable of using this technology, traditional paperwork can be electronically captured and transmitted wirelessly to receiving facilities.

Medical directors should be closely involved in the selection and purchase of medical equipment. It will be important for the medical director to stay abreast of innovations, both positive and negative, and can expect to be approached by equipment vendors and providers with requests to introduce the latest devices and technology into practice. The medical director will need to carefully review and evaluate these recommendations as often as the requests may be made in advance of evidence-based information or criteria.

Medication Supply and Storage Practices

Medications are administered to patients by EMS providers in accordance with their agency protocols and standing orders. The process in which EMS agencies receive, store, and exchange their medications will vary due to many factors such as EMS agency type (e.g., governmental, private, hospital-based, etc.), agency or regional pharmaceutical agreements, and related State and Federal regulations. Listed below are a few examples of the different processes for medication supply, storage, and exchange. The example list is not intended to describe all the various processes an EMS agency may use for this need:

- Agreement with a hospital pharmacy to provide and exchange EMS medications without any cost to the EMS agency. In these scenarios, the hospital pharmacy provides the initial stock for the EMS medications and exchanges the medications used.

- Agreement with a hospital pharmacy that EMS is billed for their initial medication inventory. Exchange of medications will occur at the receiving hospital(s).

- EMS agency will perform their own purchase, storage, and exchange of their medications.

Regardless of the process used by an EMS agency, the medical director must be knowledgeable on all related local, regional, State, and Federal regulations and requirements that affect their EMS agency's medication supply and storage practices.

If an EMS agency purchases, stores, and/or exchanges their own medications, the medical director may be responsible for enabling the agency to obtain equipment and medications. The medical director's State license will allow the EMS agency to obtain medications such as atropine, dextrose, and epinephrine. Scheduled medications such as morphine, fentanyl, and midazolam must be purchased using a prescribing number issued by the Drug Enforcement Agency (DEA). Medical directors may not use their personal DEA number to provide an EMS agency stock of controlled substances. Personal provider DEA numbers may only be used when prescribing to a specific patient. A medical director will need to obtain a separate DEA number for their EMS agency duties to avoid possible conflicts with the physician's practice. Medical directors can obtain a DEA number by completing an online application or download the forms from the following website at: www.deadiversion.usdoj.gov/drugreg/reg_apps/

The medical director must understand all State and Federal licensing requirements related to this activity. Numerous administrative and operational policies will need to be implemented to comply with all State and Federal regulations regarding medication ordering, storage, and exchange. Samplings of administrative and operational policies are listed below:

- Appropriate licensing of the EMS facility for storage of medications. To obtain licensing, numerous administrative and operational policies related to facility security, inventory security, storage parameters, and recordkeeping will need to be in place.

- Selection of a pharmaceutical vendor and compliance with medication ordering regulations.

- Requirement for recordkeeping, inventory practices, and diversion reporting for all medications.

- Requirement for documentation and process for wastage/disposal of controlled medications.

- Patient care documentation related to medication administration.

Moving Forward as a Medical Director

No emergency medical services (EMS) medical director should feel isolated and without the support of peers and other dedicated resources. Networking with medical directors of neighboring agencies is an invaluable and readily available resource. In addition, medical directors are urged to seek out additional logistical support and educational opportunities from the various regional, State, and national governmental agencies and national professional organizations listed within this handbook and its appendices.

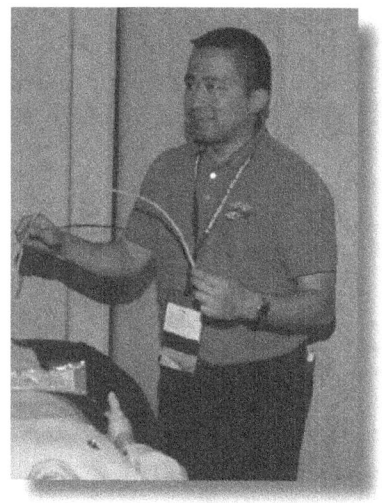

This handbook is intended to provide a reasonable overview of those fundamental issues that regularly impact the medical director operating at the EMS agency level. EMS, in the United States, represents a dynamic and diverse reality molded by local necessities, regional logistics, and State and national regulations. For this reason, it is safe to say that no two EMS agencies are the same. A medical director needs to understand the basic concepts presented here and then adapt them to both their own needs and the needs of their EMS agency. It is only through thoughtful observations, frank conversations, and committed involvement with the agency's leadership and personnel, that the medical director will be able to fully understand the dynamics of the agency and optimize their role as a medical director.

After settling into the role of medical director, the joys of shared values with EMS providers, leading and assisting with your agency's continued medical service delivery development and refinement, and making a valuable and valued contribution to the community become as important as the medicine.

Appendix A: Checklist for the New Medical Director

- ❏ Ensure affiliation agreement is reasonable with particular attention to expectations, organizational support, liability coverage, and time expectations.

- ❏ Have affiliation agreement reviewed by independent legal and tax advisors.

- ❏ Negotiate final affiliation agreement.

- ❏ Agency orientation with emergency medical services (EMS) Command Staff members.

- ❏ Meet with your agency leaders and develop strategic planning.

- ❏ Learn about dispatch practices and the Public Safety Answering Point (PSAP).

- ❏ Attend provider training drills.

- ❏ Attend agency orientation sessions.

- ❏ Shadow outgoing medical director, if possible.

- ❏ Become familiar with your EMS oversight agencies (State, regional, and local).

- ❏ Establish a comprehensive bottom-up quality management program that includes provider peer review activities with guidance by the medical director and explicit support from the agency's leadership.

- ❏ Respond and ride-along with EMS personnel to gain an understanding of capabilities, challenges, and opportunities for improvement for your providers. Do not operate in a vacuum. Be involved and engaged.

- ❏ Train with EMS providers in the areas of confined space, trench rescue, extrication, and hazmat operations in order to develop or revise specialized EMS protocols and standing orders for your agency.

- ❏ Initiate networking relationships with other medical directors in your region.

- ❏ Attend appropriate National and State conferences and meetings to network with other medical directors.

- ❏ Open lines of communications with receiving hospitals and local medical society.

- ❏ Orientation with personal protective equipment (PPE), communication equipment, and other agency-issued supplies.

Note: Seek out advice of EMS leadership for the completion of this list.

Appendix B: Glossary

Advanced Cardiac Life Support (ACLS)—A course that is taught by the American Heart Association (AHA). The course uses algorithms to educate and enhance provider skills in treating victims of cardiac arrest or other cardiopulmonary emergencies.

Advanced Emergency Medical Technician (AEMT)—This individual provides basic and limited advanced emergency medical care and transportation for patients. The AEMT has completed additional training in airway management, intravenous and/or intraosseous fluid administration, and specific emergency care medications and clinical procedures. The AEMT performs interventions with the basic and limited advanced equipment typically found on an ambulance.

Advanced Life Support (ALS)—All basic life support measures, plus invasive medical procedures including intravenous therapy, cardiac defibrillation, administration of medications and solutions, use of ventilation devices, and other procedures by State law and permitted by the medical director.

Ambulance—A vehicle designed and operated for transportation of ill and injured persons, equipped and staffed to provide for first aid or life support measures to be applied during transportation.

American College of Emergency Physicians (ACEP)—Organization of physicians associated with emergency medicine. ACEP is a leader in the development of position statements relating to emergency medical services (EMS) and trauma issues. In addition, the College develops guidelines to assist in the implementation of the position statements (e.g., Trauma Care System Guidelines). ACEP publishes the Annals of Emergency Medicine.

Automatic External Defibrillator (AED)—A device that administers an electric shock through the chest wall to the heart using built-in computers to assess the patient's heart rhythm and defibrillate as needed. Audible and/or visual prompts guide the user through the process.

Basic Life Support (BLS)—Generally limited to airway maintenance, ventilation (breathing) support, cardiopulmonary resuscitation (CPR), AED use, hemorrhage control, splinting of fractures, and management of spinal injury, protection, and transportation of the patient with accepted procedures.

Benchmarking—The process of comparing one's business processes and performance metrics to industry bests and/or best practices from other industries. Dimensions that are typically measured include quality, time, and cost.

Body Substance Isolation (BSI)—Specific steps taken to help minimize exposure to a patient's blood and other body fluids. Examples are the wearing of protective gloves, mask, gown, and eyewear.

Chain of Command—The orderly line of authority within the ranks of the incident management organization.

Collective Bargaining—Method of determining wages, hours, and other conditions of employment through direct negotiations between the union and the employer. Normally, the result of collective bargaining is a written contract that covers all employees in the bargaining unit, both union members and nonmembers.

Collective Agreement—A contract (collective agreement and contract are used interchangeably) between the union acting as the bargaining agent and the employer, covering wages, hours of work, working conditions, benefits, rights of workers and union, and procedures to be followed in settling disputes and grievances.

Commission on Accreditation of Ambulance Services (CAAS)—A private organization established to set and assist providers in maintaining the highest standards of performance in their communities. This voluntary accreditation process includes a comprehensive self-assessment and an independent, outside review of the EMS organization.

Deployment—The procedures by which ambulances are distributed throughout the service area. Deployment includes the locations and number of ambulances that are in service for a particular time period.

Emergency Medical Responder (EMR)—Formally called First Responder, is the first individual to provide emergency care at an emergency scene. This term refers to a prehospital provider who has completed training and is certified to perform basic interventions with minimal equipment.

Emergency Medical Dispatcher (EMD)—A call-taker/dispatcher at a Public Safety Answering Point (PSAP) that is specifically trained to obtain medical information from the caller over the phone and assure the dispatch of appropriate EMS resources to a given call.

Emergency Medical Services (EMS)—The provision of services to patients with medical emergencies. The purpose of EMS is to reduce the incidence of preventable injuries and illnesses, and to minimize the physical and emotional impact of injuries and illnesses. The EMS field derives its origins and body of scientific knowledge from the related fields of medicine, public health, health-care system administration, and public safety.

Emergency Medical Services Act of 1973—This act defined an EMS system as one "which provides for the arrangement of personnel, facilities, and equipment for the effective and coordinated delivery in an appropriate geographical area of health care services under emergency conditions (occurring either as a result of the patient's condition or of natural disasters or similar situations) and which is administered by a public or nonprofit private entity which has the authority and the resources to provide effective administration of the system." This act further defined components of an EMS agency as manpower, training, communications, transportation, emergency facilities, critical care units, public safety agencies, consumer participation, access to care, patient transfer, standardized recordkeeping, public information and education, agency review and evaluation, disaster planning, and mutual aid.

Emergency Medical Services (EMS) Agency—A comprehensive, coordinated arrangement of resources and functions that are organized and prepared to respond in a timely, staged manner to targeted medical emergencies, regardless of cause, in an effort to minimize the physical and emotional impact of an emergency.

Emergency Medical Technician (EMT)—This individual possesses the basic knowledge and skills necessary to provide patient care and transportation. EMTs perform interventions with the basic equipment typically found on an ambulance.

Incident Commander (IC)—The individual responsible for the management of all incident operations, including the development of strategies and both the ordering and release of resources. This individual has the authority and responsibility for conducting incident operations and is responsible for all incident operations at the incident site.

Incident Command System (ICS)—The common organizational structure for facilities, equipment, personnel, procedures, and communications at a fire department response; in an ICS, responsibility for the management of assigned resources to effectively accomplish stated objectives pertaining to an incident.

Infrastructure—The basic facilities, equipment, services, and installations needed for functioning.

International Association of EMS Chiefs (IAEMSC)—The IAEMSC is a professional association established to support, promote, and advance the leadership of response entities and to advocate for the EMS profession.

Local Government—A designation that is given to all units of government in the United States below the State level.

National Association of EMS Physicians (NAEMSP)—Organization representing physicians dedicated to prehospital emergency medical care.

National Emergency Medical Service Advisory Council (NEMSAC)—The NEMSAC is a Federal advisory committee that provides National Highway Traffic Safety Administration (NHTSA) and the Department of Transportation (DOT) advice and recommendations from nongovernmental organizations and people on a range of EMS-related issues.

National Association of Emergency Medical Technicians (NAEMT)—The national professional organization for EMTs and EMT-Paramedics. NAEMT's goals include promoting the professional status of the EMT, supporting EMS agencies at all levels, and offering guidance in current concepts of emergency medical care and government policies related to the control, certification, and licensure of EMTs.

National Emergency Medical Services Information System (NEMSIS)—A national database and data definition dictionary for the uniform collection of EMS information.

National Fire Protection Association (NFPA)—The mission of the international nonprofit NFPA, established in 1896, is to reduce the worldwide burden of fire and other hazards on the quality of life by providing and advocating consensus codes and standards, research, training, and education. The world's leading advocate of fire prevention and an authoritative source on public safety, NFPA develops, publishes, and disseminates more than 300 consensus codes and standards intended to minimize the possibility and effects of fire and other risks.

National Highway Traffic Safety Administration (NHTSA)—The agency under the DOT responsible for preventing motor vehicle injuries. NHTSA's Office of EMS conducts research and demonstration projects, distributes state-of-the-art information, provides onsite technical assistance to States and national organizations, conducts national meetings and workshops on EMS issues, supports the development of national consensus EMS standards, and serves as liaison to national EMS/trauma organizations.

National Institutes of Health (NIH)—This branch under the Public Health Service of the Department of Health and Human Services (HHS) is responsible for promoting the Nation's health through research that may be conducted by NIH researchers or simply funded by NIH.

National Registry of EMTs (NREMT)—The NREMT was founded in 1970 as the result of a task force of the American Medical Association (AMA) to provide a national EMT certification process.

Offline Medical Direction—Consists of standing orders, training, and supervision that are authorized by the medical director. All EMS providers must follow the protocols developed and/or implemented by the medical director of their EMS agency.

Online Medical Direction—The medical direction provided to out-of-hospital providers by the medical director or designee, generally in an emergency situation, either onscene or by direct voice communication. The mechanism for this contact may be radio, telephone, or other means as technology develops, but must include person-to-person communication of patient status and orders to be carried out.

Paramedic—This individual possesses the complex knowledge and skills necessary to provide advanced patient care and transportation. Paramedics have completed advanced training in all ALS procedures perform interventions with the basic and advanced equipment typically found on an ambulance.

Personal Protective Equipment (PPE)—Equipment used to protect the rescuer or EMS provider against injury or illness. Gowns, gloves, facemask, eye protection, helmet, turnout gear, protective footware, or any other protective gear to maximize the emergency providers' safety during an incident or prehospital operation.

Protocol—A set of written rules that are to be followed by EMS providers. Protocols define the total prehospital care plan for management of specific patient problems. Prehospital personnel may be authorized in advance, and in writing, to perform portions of a protocol without specific online instruction from a physician. These preauthorized treatments within a protocol are referred to as standing orders.

Provider—An individual who is certified to provide prehospital care.

Public Education—Imparts knowledge or training in specific skills. For example, teaching CPR, how to call for help properly, bicycle safety, or briefing public officials about the importance of your service to the community are all public education activities.

Public Information—The facts about an issue of public concern or a major incident in the community, or routine communications about upcoming events or presentations on annual budgets and projected needs, would all be considered public information.

Public Relations—The process of shaping public opinion through informational and educational activities.

Public Safety Answering Point (PSAP)—A call center responsible for answering calls to an emergency telephone number for police, firefighting, and EMS.

Public Utility Model (PUM)—A regulated-monopoly ambulance agency that selects the exclusive provider based on a competitive procurement process. These systems are usually tiered, providing emergency and nonemergency service with an all-ALS fleet. Commonly, a quasigovernment entity supervises the contract and performs billing and collection services.

Quality Improvement (QI)—The sum of all activities undertaken to continuously examine and improve the products and services. QI activities are described as being prospective, concurrent, or retrospective, depending on when they are conducted relative to an event (e.g., a call for prehospital medical care).

Request for Proposal (RFP)—A concise document outlining the requirements of the local government entity and allowing respondents to propose systems that would meet these requirements with cost being one factor among many. In some situations, the RFP may allow for certain postbid modifications during a final negotiated process.

Scope of Practice—Establishes what procedures a certified or licensed EMS provider is authorized to perform.

Standard of Care—The basis for evaluating a claim of negligence. The standard of care is determined by what a reasonable, prudent EMS provider of similar training, skills, and experience would do in like circumstances.

Standing Orders—See Protocol.

System Status Management (SSM)—A management tool using past service demand to predict future EMS call volume and location.

Appendix C: EMS Acronyms

AAA	American Ambulance Association
ACEP	American College of Emergency Physicians
ACLS	Advanced Cardiac Life Support
AEMT	Advanced Emergency Medical Technician
ALS	Advanced Life Support
AHA	American Heart Association
ANSI	American National Standards Institute
ATLS	Advanced Trauma Life Support
BLS	Basic Life Support
BSI	Body Substance Isolation
CAAS	Commission on Accreditation of Ambulance Services
CMS	Centers for Medicare and Medicaid Services
DHS	Department of Homeland Security
DOT	Department of Transportation
EMD	Emergency Medical Dispatcher
EMR	Emergency Medical Responder
EMS	Emergency Medical Services
EMSC	EMS for Children
EMT	Emergency Medical Technician
EVOC	Emergency Vehicle Operator Course
FEMA	Federal Emergency Management Agency
HAZMAT	Hazardous Material
HHS	Department of Health and Human Services
HIPAA	Health Insurance Portability and Accountability Act of 1996
IAEMSC	International Association of EMS Chiefs
IAFC	International Association of Fire Chiefs
IAFF	International Association of Fire Fighters
ICS	Incident Command System

ITLS	International Trauma Life Support
NAEMSE	National Association of EMS Educators
NASEMSO	National Association of State EMS Officials
NAEMSP	National Association of EMS Physicians
NAEMT	National Association of Emergency Medical Technicians
NEMSAC	National Emergency Medical Service Advisory Council
NEMSIS	National Emergency Medical Services Information System
NEMSMA	National EMS Management Association
NFFF	National Fallen Firefighters Foundation
NFPA	National Fire Protection Association
NHTSA	National Highway Traffic Safety Administration
NIMS	National Incident Management System
NIOSH	National Institute for Occupational Safety and Health
NREMT	National Registry of EMTs
NVFC	National Volunteer Fire Council
OSHA	Occupational Safety and Health Administration
PALS	Pediatric Advanced Life Support
PHTLS	Prehospital Trauma Life Support
PPE	Personal Protective Equipment
PSAP	Public Safety Answering Point
USAR	Urban Search and Rescue
USFA	U.S. Fire Administration
WMD	Weapon of Mass Destruction

Appendix D: Sample Organization Charts

Prince William County (VA) Department of Fire and Rescue
Single Agency Example

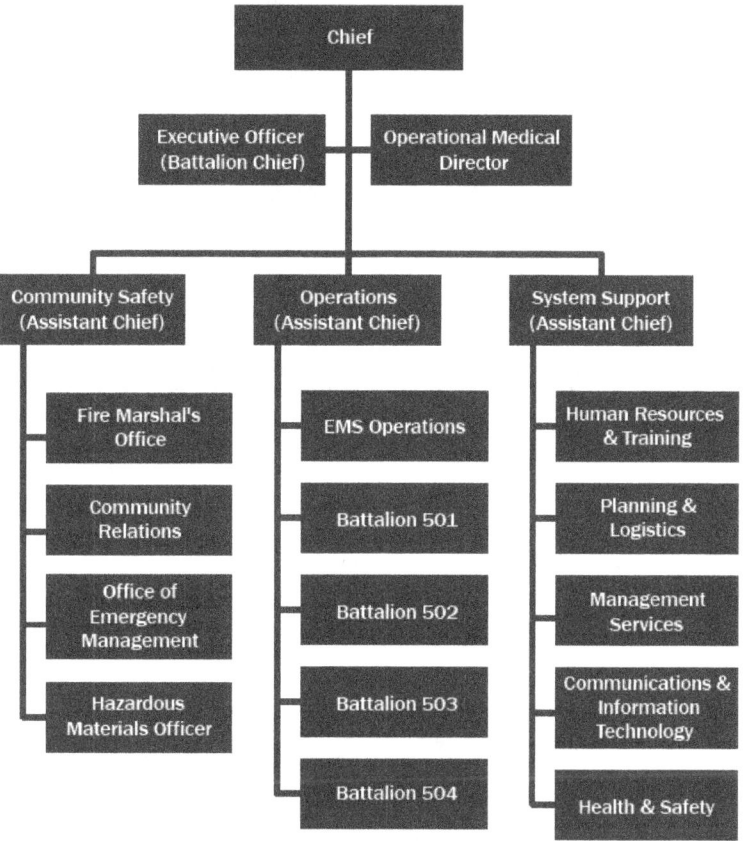

Prince William County (VA) Fire and Rescue Association
Combination System Example (12 EMS Agencies)

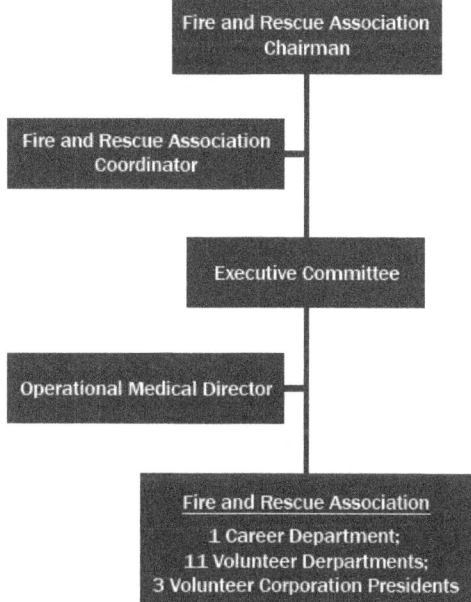

Memphis (TN) Fire Department
Single Agency Example

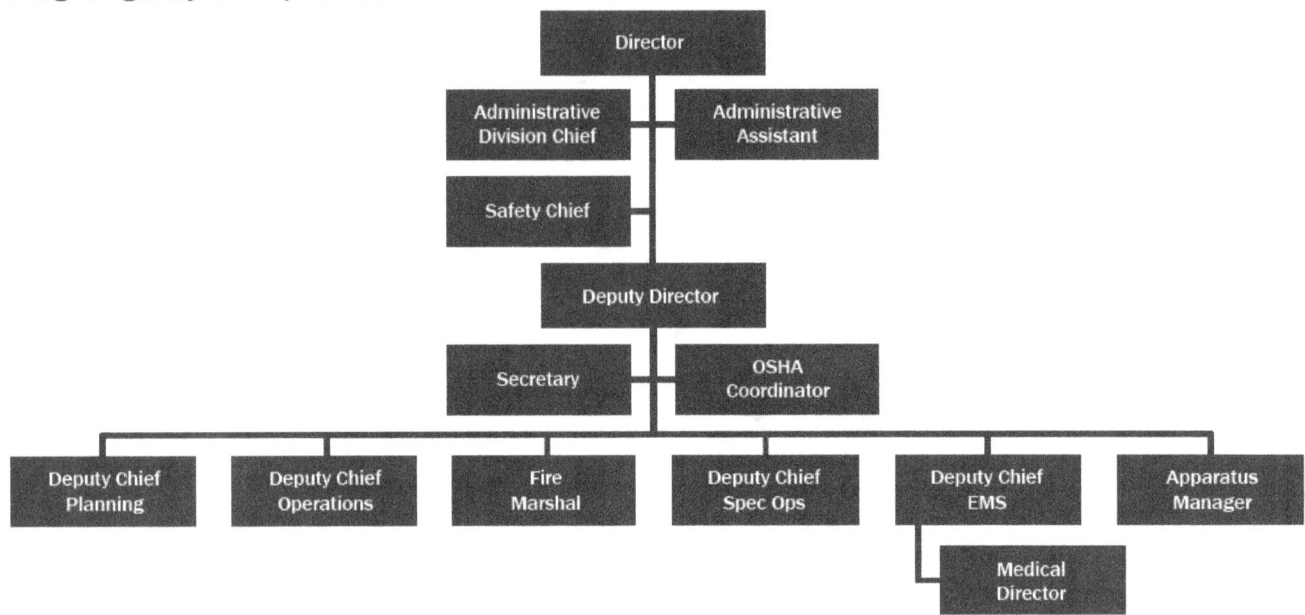

Montgomery County (MD) Fire and Rescue Service
Combination System Example

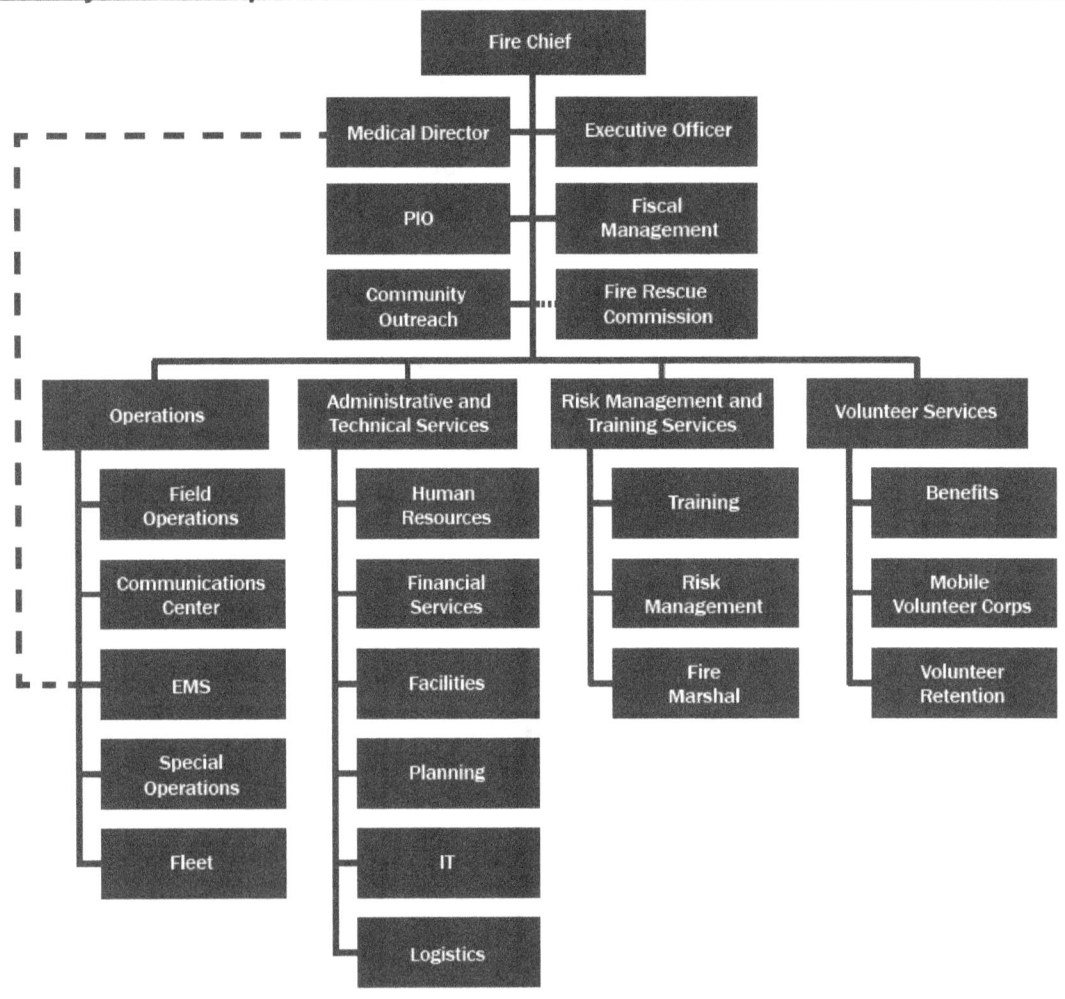

Town of Colonie (NY), Department of Emergency Medical Services
Third Service System

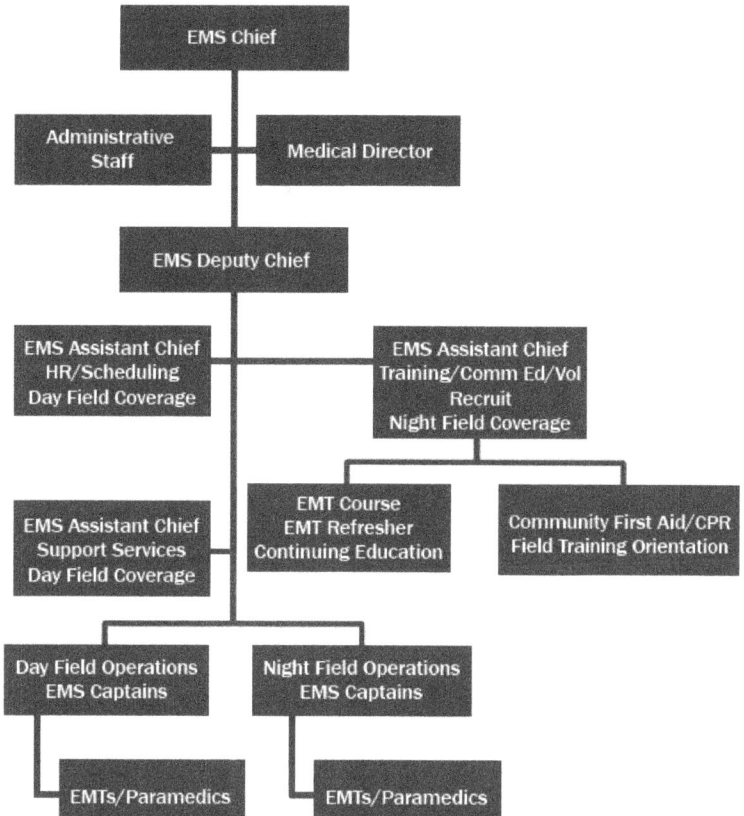

LifeCare Medical Transports (VA)
Private Ambulance (For Profit) Agency Example

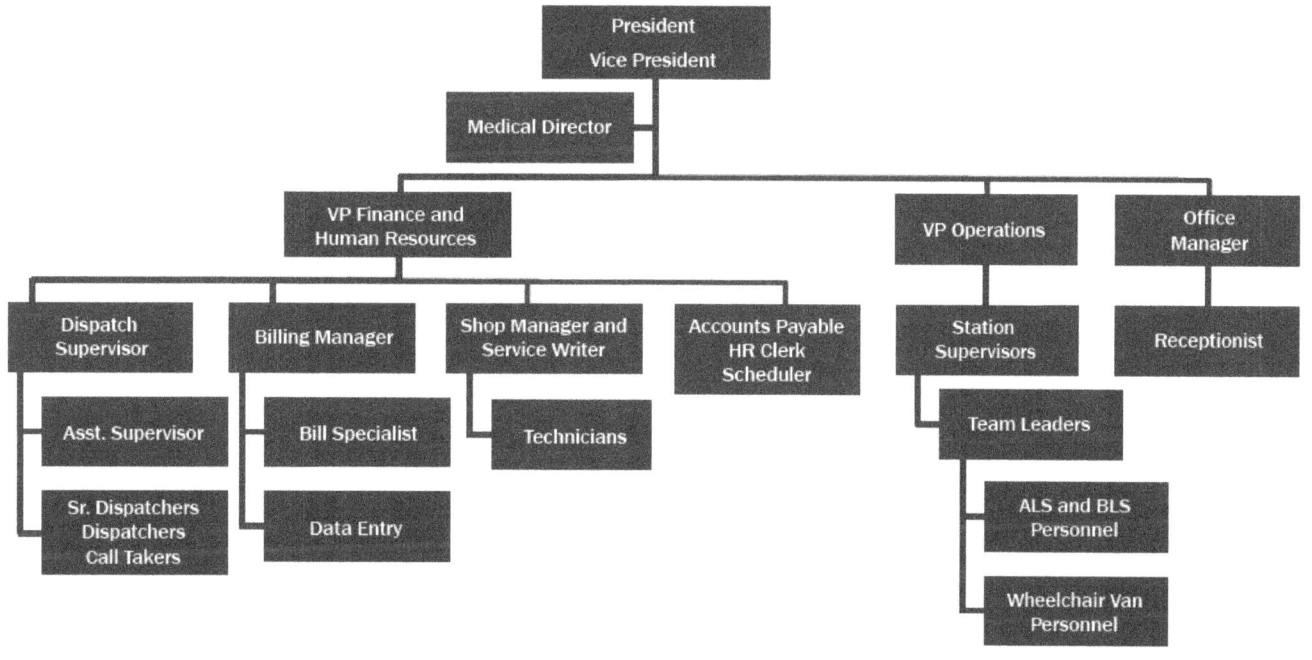

Area Metropolitan Ambulance Authority, d/b/a MedStar (TX)
Public Utility Model Agency Example

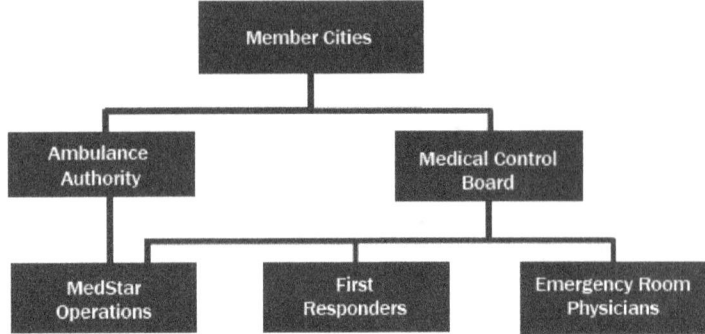

Appendix E: Sample Affiliation Agreement

AGREEMENT

This agreement made this (date) the day of, (year) by and between (agency name) hereinafter called (name) and (name), M.D., (address), hereinafter called the "Contractor."

ARTICLE 1
BASIC AGREEMENTS

1.1. SCOPE OF SERVICES. The Contractor will serve as the (agency name) EMS Medical Director throughout the term of this Agreement. As the (agency name) EMS Medical Director, Contractor will:

A. Provide off-line medical direction services to include specification, review, and approval of the service protocols, quality improvement reviews, personnel evaluations for clinical fitness for duty/coverage by medical malpractice, advice to (agency name) EMS regarding EMS and medical direction, and other mutually agreed upon duties.

B. Review reports and run sheets for incidents.

C. Assist the EMS Director in setting up and evaluating a continuous quality improvement program in accordance with the state and federal regulations.

D. Participate in educational programs for (agency name) EMS.

E. Advise the EMS Director and the County (position title) on issues relating to the provision of quality emergency medical care by the agency's personnel.

F. Assist in the planning and implementation of new/expanded programs that promote the public welfare and the welfare of the agency's personnel.

G. Provide other medical advisory services related to the first responder program and other programs of the agency as necessary.

H. Assist in the coordination of research projects and their implementation to include the obtaining of grants.

1.2. TERM. This Agreement shall commence on (date) and expires on (date).

1.3. COMPENSATION. For the satisfactory performance of the duties enumerated above, (agency name) EMS shall pay Contractor the sum of (amount) per year; said amount shall be paid in twelve (12) equal monthly payments of (amount) each, payable by the 15th day of the month after services are rendered.

1.4. EFFECT OF CONTRACTOR'S DEATH. This Agreement shall terminate immediately upon the death of the Contractor, and upon the happening of that event, the agency shall not be liable for any payments under this Agreement occurring thereafter.

ARTICLE 2
HOLD HARMLESS AND INDEMNIFICATION

Contractor shall defend, indemnify and hold harmless (agency name) EMS, its agents and employees, and (jurisdiction) County, (State) from any and all liability and expenses to Contractor or any third parties for claims, personal injuries, property damage, or loss of life or property resulting from, or in any way connected with, or alleged to have arisen from, the performance of this agreement, except where the proximate cause of such injury, damage, or loss was the sole negligence of (agency name) EMS, its agents or employees.

The Contractor shall defend, indemnify and hold (agency name) EMS, its agents and employees, and (jurisdiction) County, (state) harmless and pay all judgments that shall be rendered in any such actions, suits, claims or demands against same alleging liability referenced above, except where the proximate cause of such injury, damage or loss was the sole negligence of (agency name) EMS, its agents or employees, and (jurisdiction) County, (State).

ARTICLE 3
INSURANCE

Contractor will procure and maintain for the duration of this Agreement, Professional Liability Insurance, with a limit of not less than (amount), to cover claims for injuries to persons or damages to property which may arise from or in connection with the performance of this Agreement by the Contractor, his agents, representatives, employees or subcontractors. Additionally, Contractor will maintain automobile liability insurance for the duration of this Agreement.

ARTICLE 4
TERMINATION

Either party may cancel this Agreement, with or without cause, with a (number) day written notice to the other party. The parties are not obligated to perform or pay for any services pursuant to this Agreement after receipt of the notification of cancellation. The parties agree that this agreement is terminable at will. The parties agree that they shall not be entitled to any damages, claims, causes of action, judgment or demands in the event either party terminates this contract pursuant to this Article.

ARTICLE 5
NONDISCRIMATION

The Contractor:

5.1.   Will not discriminate against any employee or applicant for employment because of race, age, color, religion, national origin, sex or disability.

5.2.   Will take affirmative action to ensure that applicants are employed, and that employees are treated during employment, without regard to their race, age, color, religion, natural origin, sex or disability.

5.3.   Will, in all solicitations or advertisements for employees placed by or on behalf of it, state that all qualified applicants will receive consideration for employment without regard to race, age, color, religion, national origin, sex or disability.

5.4.   Will include these provisions in every subcontract or sublease let by or for him.

ARTICLE 6
ETHICAL STANDARDS

6.1.   Contractor shall not participate, directly or indirectly, through decision, approval, disapproval, recommendation, preparation of any part of a purchase request, influencing the content of any specification or purchase standard, rendering advice, investigation, auditing or otherwise, in any proceeding or application, request for ruling or other determination, claim or controversy or other matter pertaining to any contract or subcontract and any solicitation or proposal therefore, where to Contractor's knowledge there is a financial interest possessed by:

A.   The contractor or the contractor's immediate family.

B.   A business other than a public agency in which the contractor or a member of the contractor's immediate family serves as an officer, director, trustee, partner or employee.

C.   Any other person or business with whom the director or a member of contractor's immediate family is negotiating or has an arrangement concerning prospective employment.

6.2.   GRATUITIES. Contractor shall not solicit, demand, accept or agree to accept from another person or entity, anything of a pecuniary value for or because of:

A.   An official action taken, or to be taken, or which could be taken by Contractor and/or such person or entity.

B.   A legal duty performed, or to be performed, or which could be performed by Contractor and/or such person or entity.

C.   A legal duty violated, or to be violated, or which could be violated by Contractor and/or such person or entity.

6.3.   Anything of nominal value shall be presumed not to constitute a gratuity under this section.

6.4.   KICKBACKS. Contractor shall at no time receive any payment, gratuity or benefit to be made by or on behalf of a subcontractor or any person associate therewith as an inducement for the award of a subcontract or order.

ARTICLE 7
RENEWAL OF AGREEMENT

This agreement shall automatically renew for additional terms of one (number) year each unless not less than ninety (number) days from the date of termination of this agreement either party gives notice in writing to the other that such party will not renew this agreement.

ARTICLE 8
MISCELLANEOUS PROVISIONS

8.1.   Independent Contractor. The Contractor will render all services as an independent contractor; it will not be considered an employee of (agency name) EMS, nor will it be entitled to any benefits, insurance, pension, or workers' compensation as an employee of (agency name) EMS.

8.2.   Assignment. The Contractor will not assign or transfer any interest in this agreement without obtaining the prior written approval of (agency name) EMS.

8.3.   Subcontracts to the agreement. The Contractor will not enter into a subcontract for any of the services performed under this Agreement without obtaining the prior written approval of (agency name) EMS.

8.4.   Written Amendments. This Agreement may be modified only by a written amendment or addendum which has been executed and approved by the appropriate officials shown on the signature page of this Agreement.

8.5. Required Approvals. Neither the Contractor nor (agency name) EMS is bound by this Agreement until it is approved by the appropriate officials shown on the signature page of this Agreement.

8.6. Article Captions. The captions appearing in this Agreement are for convenience only and are not a part of this Agreement; they do not in any way limit or amplify the provisions of this Agreement.

8.7. Severability. If any provision of this Agreement is determined to be unenforceable or invalid, such determination will not affect the validity of the other provisions contained in this Agreement. Failure to enforce any provision of this Agreement does not affect the rights of the parties to enforce such provision in another circumstance, nor does it affect the rights of the parties to enforce any other provision of this Agreement, at any time.

8.8. Federal, State and Local Requirements. The Contractor is responsible for full compliance with all applicable federal, state and local laws, rules and regulations.

8.9. Governing Law. This Agreement will be governed and construed in accordance with the laws of the State of (name), and proper venue for litigation concerning this agreement shall be in (jurisdiction) County, (state name).

8.10. Notices. All notices of either party to terminate this agreement shall be given in writing and sent by registered mail, addressed to the other party as herein provided. Notice to (agency name) EMS shall be given at the following address: (EMS agency address); notice to the Contractor shall be given at (address).

IN WITNESS WHEREOF, the parties have executed or caused to be executed this agreement on its behalf, the date and year first above written in duplicate originals.

_____EMS

by

_____
EMS official

_____
your name

Appendix F: Sample Liability Insurance Form

ACORD®   **CERTIFICATE OF LIABILITY INSURANCE**   DATE (MM/DD/YYYY)

THIS CERTIFICATE IS ISSUED AS A MATTER OF INFORMATION ONLY AND CONFERS NO RIGHTS UPON THE CERTIFICATE HOLDER. THIS CERTIFICATE DOES NOT AFFIRMATIVELY OR NEGATIVELY AMEND, EXTEND OR ALTER THE COVERAGE AFFORDED BY THE POLICIES BELOW. THIS CERTIFICATE OF INSURANCE DOES NOT CONSTITUTE A CONTRACT BETWEEN THE ISSUING INSURER(S), AUTHORIZED REPRESENTATIVE OR PRODUCER, AND THE CERTIFICATE HOLDER.

IMPORTANT: If the certificate holder is an ADDITIONAL INSURED, the policy(ies) must be endorsed. If SUBROGATION IS WAIVED, subject to the terms and conditions of the policy, certain policies may require an endorsement. A statement on this certificate does not confer rights to the certificate holder in lieu of such endorsement(s).

PRODUCER	CONTACT NAME		
	PHONE (A/C, No, Ext):		FAX (A/C, No):
	E-MAIL ADDRESS:		
	INSURER(S) AFFORDING COVERAGE		NAIC #
	INSURER A :		
INSURED	INSURER B :		
	INSURER C :		
	INSURER D :		
	INSURER E :		
	INSURER F :		

COVERAGES   **CERTIFICATE NUMBER:**   **REVISION NUMBER:**

THIS IS TO CERTIFY THAT THE POLICIES OF INSURANCE LISTED BELOW HAVE BEEN ISSUED TO THE INSURED NAMED ABOVE FOR THE POLICY PERIOD INDICATED. NOTWITHSTANDING ANY REQUIREMENT, TERM OR CONDITION OF ANY CONTRACT OR OTHER DOCUMENT WITH RESPECT TO WHICH THIS CERTIFICATE MAY BE ISSUED OR MAY PERTAIN, THE INSURANCE AFFORDED BY THE POLICIES DESCRIBED HEREIN IS SUBJECT TO ALL THE TERMS, EXCLUSIONS AND CONDITIONS OF SUCH POLICIES. LIMITS SHOWN MAY HAVE BEEN REDUCED BY PAID CLAIMS.

INSR LTR	TYPE OF INSURANCE	ADDL INSR	SUBR WVD	POLICY NUMBER	POLICY EFF (MM/DD/YYYY)	POLICY EXP (MM/DD/YYYY)	LIMITS	
X	**GENERAL LIABILITY**						EACH OCCURRENCE	$ 1,000,000
	X COMMERCIAL GENERAL LIABILITY						DAMAGE TO RENTED PREMISES (Ea occurrence)	$ 100,000
	CLAIMS-MADE X OCCUR						MED EXP (Any one person)	$ 5,000
X	ESIP Emerg Lia						PERSONAL & ADV INJURY	$ 1,000,000
	Med Dir Malpr						GENERAL AGGREGATE	$ 10,000,000
	GEN'L AGGREGATE LIMIT APPLIES PER:						PRODUCTS - COMP/OP AGG	$ 10,000,000
	POLICY PRO-JECT LOC							$
	AUTOMOBILE LIABILITY						COMBINED SINGLE LIMIT (Ea accident)	$
	ANY AUTO						BODILY INJURY (Per person)	$
	ALL OWNED AUTOS SCHEDULED AUTOS						BODILY INJURY (Per accident)	$
	HIRED AUTOS NON-OWNED AUTOS						PROPERTY DAMAGE (Per accident)	$
								$
	UMBRELLA LIAB X OCCUR						EACH OCCURRENCE	$ 5,000,000
	EXCESS LIAB CLAIMS-MADE						AGGREGATE	$ 5,000,000
	DED X RETENTION $ 0							$
	WORKERS COMPENSATION AND EMPLOYERS' LIABILITY Y/N						WC STATU-TORY LIMITS OTH-ER	
	ANY PROPRIETOR/PARTNER/EXECUTIVE OFFICER/MEMBER EXCLUDED? (Mandatory in NH)	N/A					E.L. EACH ACCIDENT	$
							E.L. DISEASE - EA EMPLOYEE	$
	If yes, describe under DESCRIPTION OF OPERATIONS below						E.L. DISEASE - POLICY LIMIT	$

DESCRIPTION OF OPERATIONS / LOCATIONS / VEHICLES (Attach ACORD 101, Additional Remarks Schedule, if more space is required)

CERTIFICATE HOLDER	CANCELLATION
	SHOULD ANY OF THE ABOVE DESCRIBED POLICIES BE CANCELLED BEFORE THE EXPIRATION DATE THEREOF, NOTICE WILL BE DELIVERED IN ACCORDANCE WITH THE POLICY PROVISIONS.
	AUTHORIZED REPRESENTATIVE

© 1988-2010 ACORD CORPORATION. All rights reserved.

ACORD 25 (2010/05)   The ACORD name and logo are registered marks of ACORD

Appendix G: Industry Regulations and Standards

Occupational Safety and Health Administration

The two Occupational Safety and Health Administration (OSHA) regulations that govern emergency medical services (EMS) are found at Title 29 CFR § 1910.120: *Occupational Safety and Health Standards*; subparts (q)(6) (Hazardous waste operations and emergency response; and emergency response to hazardous substance releases). Each regulation deals with the level of responsibilities that EMS personnel have when responding to incidents involving hazardous substances, as well as the *Hazardous Waste Operations and Emergency Response* (HAZWOPER) training required.

The States and jurisdictions operating under OSHA covering both the private sector and State and local government employees are

- Alaska
- Arizona
- California
- Connecticut
- Hawaii
- Illinois
- Indiana

- Iowa
- Kentucky
- Maryland
- Michigan
- Minnesota
- Nevada
- New Mexico

- New Jersey
- New York
- North Carolina
- Oregon
- Puerto Rico
- South Carolina
- Tennessee

- Utah
- Vermont
- Virgin Islands
- Virginia
- Washington
- Wyoming

National Fire Protection Association

National Fire Protection Association (NFPA) 450, *Guide for Emergency Medical Services and Systems*, requires the coordination and cooperation of disparate elements. NFPA 450 is a document created to assist individuals, agencies, organizations, or systems, as well as those interested or involved in emergency medical services (EMS) agency design. It presents a practical framework of specific guidelines and recommendations that can be used to design and/or evaluate a comprehensive EMS agency.

NFPA 1500, *Standard on Fire Department Occupational Safety and Health Program*, addresses occupational safety in the working environment of the fire service and safety in the proper use of fire department vehicles, tools, equipment, protective clothing, and protective breathing apparatus.

NFPA 1584, *Standard on the Rehabilitation Process for Members During Emergency Operations and Training Exercises*, provides for an organized approach for fire department members' rehabilitation during emergency operations and training exercises should be an integral component of both an occupational safety and health program and incident scene management. Document reflects current science and knowledge on rehabilitation of fire service members.

NFPA 1710, *Standard for the Organization and Deployment of Fire Suppression Operations, Emergency Medical Operations, and Special Operations to the Public by Career Fire Departments*, identifies the minimum requirements related to the organization and deployment of fire suppression operations, emergency medical operations, and special operations to the public by substantially all career fire departments.

NFPA 1720, *Standard for the Organization and Deployment of Fire Suppression Operations, Emergency Medical Operations and Special Operations to the Public by Volunteer Fire Departments*, identifies the minimum requirements relating to the organization and deployment of fire suppression operations, emergency medical operations, and special operations to the public by volunteer and combination fire departments.

Dependent of the specialized functions an agency may provide, the following NFPA standards may be of additional interest to the medical director:

- NFPA 72, *National Fire Alarm Code;*

- NFPA 471, *Recommended Practice for Responding to Hazardous Materials Incidents;*

- NFPA 472, *Standard for Competence of Responders to Hazardous Materials/Weapons of Mass Destruction Incidents;*

- NFPA 473, *Standard for Competencies for EMS Personnel Responding to Hazardous Materials/Weapons of Mass Destruction Incidents;*

- NFPA 1026, *Standard for Incident Management Personnel Professional Qualifications;*

- NFPA 1051, *Standard for Wildland Fire Fighter Professional Qualifications;*

- NFPA 1143, *Standard for Wildland Fire Management;*

- NFPA 1221, *Standard for the Installation, Maintenance, and Use of Emergency Services Communications Systems;*

- NFPA 1404, *Standard for Fire Service Respiratory Protection Training;*

- NFPA 1582, *Standard on Comprehensive Occupational Medical Program for Fire Departments;*

- NFPA 1583, *Standard on Health-Related Fitness Programs for Fire Department Members;*

- NFPA 1600, *Standard on Disaster/Emergency Management and Business Continuity Programs;*

- NFPA 1670, *Standard on Operations and Training for Technical Search and Rescue Incidents;*

- NFPA 1917, *Standard for Automotive Ambulances;* and

- NFPA 1999, *Standard on Protective Clothing for Emergency Medical Operations.*

American Society for Testing and Materials

The American Society for Testing and Materials (ASTM) International produces several standards related to EMS, the medical director, and emergency medical dispatcher (EMD). A sampling of standards is

- F1149-93 (2008), *Standard Practice for Qualifications, Responsibilities, and Authority of Individuals and Institutions Providing Medical Direction of Emergency Medical Services;*

- F1258-95 (2006), *Standard Practice for Emergency Medical Dispatch;*

- F1552-94 (2009), *Standard Practice for Training Instructor Qualification and Certification Eligibility of Emergency Medical Dispatchers;* and

- F1560-00 (2006), *Standard Practice for Emergency Medical Dispatch Management.*

Appendix H: Performance Measures

EMS Agency Performance Measures at a Glance: Example from International Association of Fire Fighters (IAFF)

Indicator	Definition of Indicator	Rationale Relating Measure to Agency Quality	Established Standard	Measure Type	Measure Status	Performance Goal	Performance Measure	Data Element Source
Call Processing	Time from call intake by dispatch agency until unit notification including answering phone (alarm), gathering vital information, and initiating a response by dispatching appropriate units.	Communication and dispatch component play major role in efficiency, agency deployment, and response. Communications component must be measured to assess individual operations quality.	NFPA 1221	Process	Core	95% of calls processed in less that 90 seconds	2.1 What percentage of all EMS calls is processed by the agency actually dispatching the responding unit in 90 seconds or less?	Dispatch Log, recorded communication archives, Dispatch administrator.
Turnout Time	Time from response unit notification to vehicle wheels rolling toward incident location. Includes personnel preparation for response, boarding responding apparatus/vehicle, placing the apparatus/vehicle in gear for response, wheels rolling toward the emergency scene.	The time from alert to wheels turning provides an indication of the state of readiness of personnel. Minimizing this time is crucial to an immediate response.	NFPA 1710	Process	Core	90% of all calls turned out in less than 60 seconds	2.2 What percentage of all EMS calls is turned out in 60 seconds or less?	Dispatch logs, Response Unit Station log, Recorded Communication Archives, Call reports.
Response Time	Timer from responding vehicle wheels rolling toward the address/incident until the arrival of the vehicle on scene at that address/incident location.	This measurement is indicative of the agency's capability to adequately staff, locate, and deploy response resources. It is also indicative of responding personnel's knowledge of the area or dispatcher instruction for efficient travel.	NFPA 1710	Process	Core	a. First responder with minimum of BLS capability = 90% in 4 minutes. b. Transport capable vehicle = 90% in 8 minutes. c. ALS capability = 90% in 8 minutes.	2.3a. What percentage of all EMS calls achieve first responding unit travel time of 4 minutes 0 seconds or less? 2.3b. What percentage of all EMS calls achieve transport unit travel time of 8 minutes 0 seconds or less? 2.3c. What percentage of all EMS call achieve ALS unit travel time of 8 minutes 0 seconds or less? 2.3d. Does the agency use Agency Status Management?	Dispatch logs, response Unit Station log, Computerized/Recorded Communications Archive, Call documentation reports.

EMS Agency Performance Measures at a Glance: Example from International Association of Fire Fighters (IAFF) (continued)

Indicator	Definition of Indicator	Rationale Relating Measure to Agency Quality	Established Standard	Measure Type	Measure Status	Performance Goal	Performance Measure	Data Element Source
Staffing	The indicator includes both the number and level of training of personnel deployed on an emergency call.	The level of training of personnel deployed is indicative of the quality of the services delivered and therefore the agency. Anecdotally, two or more advanced personnel are considered higher quality than one.	NFPA 1710	Process	Core	Compliance with State regulations for staffing ALS transport units. Compliance with NFPA 1710 standards for staffing ALS response units.	2.4a. What percentage of ALS level calls receives a response including two EMTs and two paramedics? 2.4b. What percentage of BLS level calls receives a response including two EMTs?	Standard Operating Procedures (SOPs), Departmental Policy, Staffing Records.

Outcome-centered example from Myers et al. Prehosp Emerg Care. 2008; 12(2):141-51.

(www.ncbi.nlm.nih.gov/pubmed/18379908)

Complaint/Disease process	Indicators
ST-segment elevation myocardial infarction (STEMI)	• Aspirin administered (if not allergic) • 12-lead electrocardiogram (ECG) performed with direct activation of interventional cardiology team • Direct transport to facility capable of emergent percutaneous coronary interventions
Pulmonary edema	• Nitroglycerin administered (if no contraindications) • Continuous positive airway pressure (CPAP) attempted before endotracheal intubation
Asthma	• Beta-agonist administered
Seizure	• Blood glucose measured • Benzodiazepine administered for status epilepticus
Trauma	• Scene time limited to <10 minutes (excluding entrapped time) • Direct transport to trauma center (or transfer to air transport) for patients meeting criteria
Cardiac arrest	• Response interval for CPR and defibrillator <5 minutes

Appendix I: Endnotes

[1] National Highway Traffic Safety Administration (NHTSA). 1996. "EMS Agenda for the Future." Washington, DC: Department of Transportation (DOT).

[2] Institute of Medicine. Committee on the Future of Emergency Care in the United States Health Agency. 2007. "Emergency Medical Services at the Crossroads." Washington, DC: National Academies Press.

[3] Eversole, J.M. 2003. *The Fire Chief's Handbook* (6th ed.). Tulsa: PennWell Corp.

[4] Ibid.

[5] National Registry of Emergency Medical Technicians—NREMT Milestones. 2008. Retrieved November 10, 2010, from website: nremt.org/nremt/about/nremtMilestones.asp

[6] Institute of Medicine. Committee on the Future of Emergency Care in the United States Health Agency. 2007. "Emergency Medical Services at the Crossroads." Washington, DC: National Academies Press.

[7] NHTSA. 1996. "EMS Agenda for the Future." Washington, DC: DOT.

[8] NHTSA. 2000. "EMS Education Agenda for the Future: A Systems Approach." Washington, DC: DOT.

[9] Institute of Medicine. Committee on the Future of Emergency Care in the United States Health Agency. 2007. "Emergency Medical Services at the Crossroads." Washington, DC: National Academies Press.

[10] Ibid.

[11] NHTSA. 2005. "National EMS Scope of Practice Model." Washington, DC: DOT.

[12] International Association of Fire Fighters (IAFF). *Emergency Medical Services: A Guidebook for Fire-Based Agencies.* (4th ed.). Retrieved April 29, 2010, from website: www.iaff.org/Tech/PDF/EMSGuideBk.pdf

[13] Institute of Medicine. Committee on the Future of Emergency Care in the United States Health Agency. 2007. "Emergency Medical Services at the Crossroads." Washington, DC: National Academies Press.

[14] Ibid.

[15] American College of Emergency Physicians. "Policy Statement: Medical Direction of Emergency Medical Services." 2005. Retrieved April 29, 2010, from website: www.acep.org/practres.aspx?id=29570

[16] National Association of EMS Physicians. 2002. "Prehospital Agency and Medical Oversight" (3rd ed.). Dubuque: Kendall/Hunt Pub. 441-460.

[17] Sanders, M.J., Lewis, L., and Quick, Gary. 2007. *Paramedic Text Book* (Rev. 3rd ed.). St. Louis, MO: Elsevier Mosby Inc.

[18] Ibid.

[19] American College of Emergency Physicians. "Policy Statement: Direction of Out-of-Hospital Care at the Scene of Medical Emergencies." Retrieved May 26, 2010, from website: www.acep.org/practres. aspx?id=29170cuments/

[20] NHTSA. "National Emergency Medical Services Educational Standards." Retrieved September 2, 2010, from website: www.ems.gov/pdf/811077a.pdf

[21] The Continuing Education Coordinating Board for Emergency Medical Services (CECBEMS). "Frequently Asked Questions." Retrieved on September 2, 2010, from website: www.cecbems.org/faqAnswers

22 NHTSA. "A Leadership Guide to Quality Improvement in Emergency Medical Services Agencies." Retrieved on May 23, 2010, from website: www.nhtsa.gov/people/injury/ems/leaderguide/index.html

23 Evans, B.E., and Dyar, J.T. 2010. "Management of EMS." Upper Saddle River, NJ: Pearson Education, Inc. 8-21.

24 National Association of State Emergency Medical Services Directors (NASEMSD), National Association of EMS Physicians (NAEMSP), and American College of Emergency Physicians (ACEP). "The Role of State Medical Direction in the Comprehensive Emergency Medical Services Agency." Retrieved on April 26, 2010, from website: www.acep.org/workarea/showcontent.aspx?id=4850

25 American Academy of Orthopedic Surgeons. 2006. "Emergency Care and Transportation of the Sick and Injured." (9th ed.). Sudbury, MA: Jones & Bartlett Publishers.

26 Dave, G., and Parmar, K. 2001. "Emergency Medical Services and Disaster Management: A Holistic Approach." (1st ed.). New Delhi, India: Jaypee Brothers Medical Publishers, Ltd.

27 Ibid.

28 Six Sigma Online. "Why Six Sigma?" Retrieved on April 22, 2011, from website: www.sixsigmaonline.org/q1.html

29 Lee County EMS. "Lee County EMS and the Implementation of Six Sigma." Retrieved on September 1, 2010, from website: home.safelee.org/public/sixsigma/

30 IAFF and International Association of Fire Chiefs (IAFC). "EMS System Performance Measurement." Retrieved on November 10, 2010, from website: www.iaff.org/tech/PDF/EMSSystemPerformanceMeasurement.pdf

31 Ibid.

32 Hatley T. "Using Data in Quality Management." NAEMSP, Vol. 3. Retrieved on September 1, 2010, from website: www.naemsp.org/newsletters.html

33 Touchstone, M. (2009, January). "EMS in America: The Foundation Documents." EMS1.com. Retrieved on August 28, 2010, from website: www.ems1.com/ems-products/education/articles/584788-EMS-in-America-The-Foundation-Documents/

34 The Commission on Accreditation of Ambulance Services (CAAS). "Welcome to CAAS." Retrieved on August 26, 2010, from website: www.caas.org/

35 Prehospital Care Research Forum. "EMS Research." Retrieved on September 4, 2010, from website: www.pcrf.mednet.ucla.edu/pcrf/pdf4.pdf

36 Federal Emergency Management Agency (FEMA). "Standard Details." 29 CFR Part 634 - Worker Visibility. Retrieved on August 31, 2010, from website: www.rkb.us/contentdetail.cfm?content_id=200622

37 Goodson, C. 2001. "Principles of Vehicle Extrication" (2nd ed.). Oklahoma City: Fire Protection Publications, Oklahoma State University.

38 Commission on Accreditation of Allied Health Education Programs. "Standards and Guidelines." Retrieved on August 26, 2010, from website: www.coaemsp.org/Documents/Standards.pdf

39 NHTSA. "EMS Workforce for the 21st Century: A National Assessment." Retrieved on August 28, 2010, from website: www.nhtsa.gov/people/injury/ems/EMSUpdateFall/pages/page5.htm

40 Kearns, C. (2007, August). "Monitor Your Budget on a Daily Basis." EMS World. Retrieved on August 28, 2010, from website: www.emsresponder.com/publication/article.jsp?pubId=1&id=6002&submit_comment=y#commentform

www.ingramcontent.com/pod-product-compliance
Lightning Source LLC
Chambersburg PA
CBHW081143170526
45165CB00008B/2773